Integrative Male Reproductive Health - Risk, Mechanisms, and Interventions

Edited by Mohammad Ishraq Zafar

Published in London, United Kingdom

Integrative Male Reproductive Health - Risk, Mechanisms, and Interventions
http://dx.doi.org/10.5772/intechopen.1008029
Edited by Mohammad Ishraq Zafar

Contributors
Abdullatif E. Al-Terki, Abdulrahman Almazeedi, Agni Pantou, Ali Almoumen, Aris Kaltsas, Athanasios Zachariou, Athanasios Zikopoulos, Atsushi Takenaka, Daniel Ionut Berean, Dimitrios Baltogiannis, Ioannis Giannakis, Maryam Albuloushi, Nan Liu, Naser Al-Soudan Al-Anazi, Nikolaos Sofikitis, Qiming Yang, Said M. Yaiesh, Shabnoor Iqbal, Sofoklis Stavros, Talal A. Alenezi, Tariq F. Al-Shaiji, Usman Mir Khan, Vladimir Kojovic, Zubair Muhammad

First published in London, United Kingdom, 2025 by IntechOpen
IntechOpen is the global imprint of INTECHOPEN LIMITED, registered in England and Wales, registration number: 11086078, 167-169 Great Portland Street, London, W1W 5PF, United Kingdom

For EU product safety concerns: IN TECH d.o.o., Prolaz Marije Krucifikse Kozulić 3, 51000 Rijeka, Croatia, info@intechopen.com or visit our website at intechopen.com.

British Library Cataloguing-in-Publication Data
A catalogue record for this book is available from the British Library

Integrative Male Reproductive Health - Risk, Mechanisms, and Interventions
Edited by Mohammad Ishraq Zafar
p. cm.
Print ISBN 978-1-83635-400-0
Online ISBN 978-1-83635-399-7
eBook (PDF) ISBN 978-1-83635-401-7

If disposing of this product, please recycle the paper responsibly.

Meet the editor

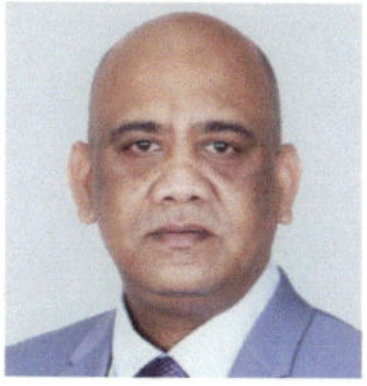

Dr. Mohammad Ishraq Zafar is a Distinguished Associate Researcher, Principal Investigator, and Post-Graduate Supervisor at the Department of Obstetrics & Gynecology, Center of Reproductive Medicine, Fourth Affiliated Hospital of School of Medicine, and International School of Medicine, International Institute of Medicine, Zhejiang University, Yiwu, P. R. China. His research focuses on endocrinology, male reproductive health, and endocrine-related infertility, with emphasis on metabolism, therapeutic interventions, and reproductive epigenetics. Dr. Zafar maintains an extensive publication record and serves in key editorial positions, including Associate Editor of Frontiers in Endocrinology (Reproductive Medicine Section), Academic Editor of PLOS ONE, and Editorial Board Member of Biomedical Reports and Medicine International journals. He is also a Chartered Scientist (CSci) and a member of the Royal Society of Biology and the European Society of Human Reproduction & Embryology.

Contents

Preface **IX**

Section 1
Environmental Challenges and Cellular Protection **1**

Chapter 1 **3**
Microplastics Exposure Is Harmful to Male Reproductive Health
by Zubair Muhammad, Qiming Yang and Nan Liu

Chapter 2 **45**
Role of Antioxidants in Male Semen Preservation
by Daniel Ionut Berean

Section 2
Clinical Management and Therapeutic Interventions **69**

Chapter 3 **71**
Urological Congenitalism, Reconstruction and Neuro-Urological Male Patients: Reproductive Health and Fertility Challenges and Their Contemporary Management
by Talal A. Alenezi, Abdulrahman Almazeedi, Maryam Albuloushi, Ali Almoumen, Naser Al-Soudan Al-Anazi, Abdullatif E. Al-Terki, Tariq F. Al-Shaiji and Said M. Yaiesh

Chapter 4 **117**
Emerging Therapies Targeting Male Reproductive Aging Processes
by Shabnoor Iqbal and Usman Mir Khan

Chapter 5 **159**
Understanding Male Sexual Function after TESE or mTESE: A Narrative Review
by Athanasios Zachariou, Ioannis Giannakis, Dimitrios Baltogiannis, Aris Kaltsas, Athanasios Zikopoulos, Sofoklis Stavros, Vladimir Kojovic, Agni Pantou, Atsushi Takenaka and Nikolaos Sofikitis

Preface

Male reproductive health has rapidly evolved into a dynamic field at the intersection of molecular biology, clinical medicine, and environmental science. Shifting demographic trends, notably delayed fatherhood, alongside advances in surgical and pharmacological innovation and recognition of emerging environmental threats, are redefining both clinical practice and research priorities. This book addresses this evolving landscape by providing an integrative overview of contemporary themes in male fertility and sexual health. It is intended to serve andrologists, reproductive endocrinologists, urologists, sexual medicine specialists, translational scientists, environmental health researchers, and trainees seeking a structured and forward-looking synthesis of male reproductive health.

The first section examines environmental challenges and cellular protection mechanisms that define contemporary reproductive health threats and responses. It presents current evidence linking exposure to ubiquitous environmental pollutants, particularly microplastics, with impaired sperm quality and potential transgenerational effects, acknowledging the methodological and regulatory challenges in exposure assessment and the establishment of causal relationships. This section further highlights oxidative stress, driven by reactive oxygen species, as a primary contributor to sperm damage and infertility, evaluating both conventional and advanced therapeutic interventions, including nanotechnology-based delivery systems, mitochondria-targeted molecules, biomarker-guided supplementation, and genetic profiling. Broader considerations, including disparities in healthcare access, fertility preservation, and cryopreservation, are also discussed.

The second section addresses clinical management and therapeutic interventions across diverse patient populations and clinical contexts. It reviews male fertility and sexual health challenges associated with congenital and neuro-urological conditions, such as cryptorchidism, bladder exstrophy, prune belly syndrome, and spinal dysraphism, as well as acquired disorders, including spinal cord injury, multiple sclerosis, and cerebrovascular disease. Management strategies include surgical interventions, such as orchiopexy, phalloplasty, prosthetic implantation, and urinary tract reconstruction, as well as assisted reproductive technologies within multidisciplinary and transitional care models. This section explores age-related reproductive decline, detailing the biology of testicular aging, reduced androgen production, and systemic consequences, contrasting established treatments with emerging strategies, including anti-inflammatory and antioxidant therapies, phosphodiesterase-5 inhibitors, nitric oxide donors, dopamine agonists, and combination approaches aimed at optimizing reproductive and systemic health. The outcomes of sperm retrieval procedures, specifically testicular sperm extraction (TESE) and microdissection TESE (Micro-TESE), are examined in the context of balancing improved retrieval rates with risks such as testosterone deficiency, erectile dysfunction, and psychological distress. Special attention is given to vulnerable subpopulations, notably men with Klinefelter syndrome, focusing on hormonal recovery and psychosocial support.

The Editor extends sincere gratitude to the contributing authors for their expertise and to Mr. Mateo Belir, Publishing Process Manager, for his dedicated support throughout the manuscript handling process.

Mohammad Ishraq Zafar
Department of Obstetrics and Gynecology,
Center for Reproductive Medicine,
Fourth Affiliated Hospital of School of Medicine,
International School of Medicine,
International Institutes of Medicine,
Zhejiang University,
Yiwu, Zhejiang, P.R. China

Section 1

Environmental Challenges and Cellular Protection

Chapter 1

Microplastics Exposure Is Harmful to Male Reproductive Health

Zubair Muhammad, Qiming Yang and Nan Liu

Abstract

This chapter will delve into the burgeoning concern surrounding microplastics (MPs) exposure and its insidious impact on male reproductive health. MPs, ubiquitous environmental pollutants stemming from the degradation of plastic products, have permeated various ecosystems and consequently found their way into the human body through multiple exposure routes, such as ingestion via food and water, and inhalation of airborne MP particles. The scope of this chapter encompasses an in-depth exploration of the mechanisms through which MPs exert their deleterious effects. It will examine the potential for MPs to induce oxidative stress in male reproductive tissues, leading to damage of sperm cells and disruption of the blood-testis barrier. Furthermore, the endocrine-disrupting properties of MPs will be scrutinized, as these pollutants can interfere with the normal hormonal regulation of the male reproductive system, affecting testosterone production and spermatogenesis. In addition, the chapter will present epidemiological evidence linking MPs exposure to adverse reproductive outcomes in men, such as reduced sperm quality, including decreased sperm count, motility, and morphology, as well as an increased risk of male infertility. Animal studies that have provided crucial insights into the dose-response relationships and the potential for transgenerational effects of MPs on male reproductive health will also be discussed. By synthesizing the existing body of knowledge, this chapter aims to highlight the urgent need for further research and public health interventions to mitigate the potential harm of MPs to male reproductive health.

Keywords: microplastics (MPs), environmental pollution, male reproductive health, public health, male fertility, semen quality

1. Introduction

The escalating dispersion of plastic pollutants has become a critical environmental crisis, threatening marine and terrestrial ecosystems while posing a potential threat to human health [1]. When exposed to environmental stressors, degradation of bulk plastics occurs into microplastics (MPs)—particulate matter $\leq$5 mm in size—that circulate through global ecosystems, including oceans, freshwater bodies, and soil. These MPs are the products of the degradation and wear and tear of different plastic products, including automobile trim, textiles, and paint coatings in addition to spills of pellets and powders during the pre-production processes.

And now, as ubiquitous in the environment, they can infiltrate the trophic chain, raising concerns due to their persistent detection in edible matrices and their capacity to bypass biological barriers. Human exposure occurs via multiple pathways: dietary intake, such as seafood [2], bottled water [3], milk, beer, and table salt [4, 5], water consumption, and inhalation of airborne particles [6]. Beyond the gastrointestinal tract, MPs have been identified in multiple organ systems, including the respiratory, circulatory [7], reproductive, nervous, immune, endocrine, urinary, and musculoskeletal systems [2, 8], suggesting broad-ranging biological interactions.

1.1 Global proliferation of MPs

Plastic pollution in marine, terrestrial ecosystems, fresh water, and the atmosphere environments is widespread and pervasive. However, the scientific community is only beginning to comprehend the interaction between environmental plastic contamination and earth's biogeochemical cycles, specifically those involving carbon, nitrogen, phosphorus, and sulfur. MPs are extensively distributed across diverse global ecosystems, including oceans, lakes, rivers, and soils. Due to their abilities to integrate into the soil and sediment matrices, MPs significantly alter the physicochemical properties, element cycling processes, and greenhouse gas emissions. Furthermore, microbial metabolism of plastics, along with dissolved organic matter derived from plastic leachates, may directly or indirectly impact critical biogeochemical pathways. Notably, the "plastisphere", defined as the assemblage of microbial communities that colonize plastic debris, is emerging as an especially important role to the cycling of essential elements (**Figure 1**) [9]. Understanding the plastisphere's

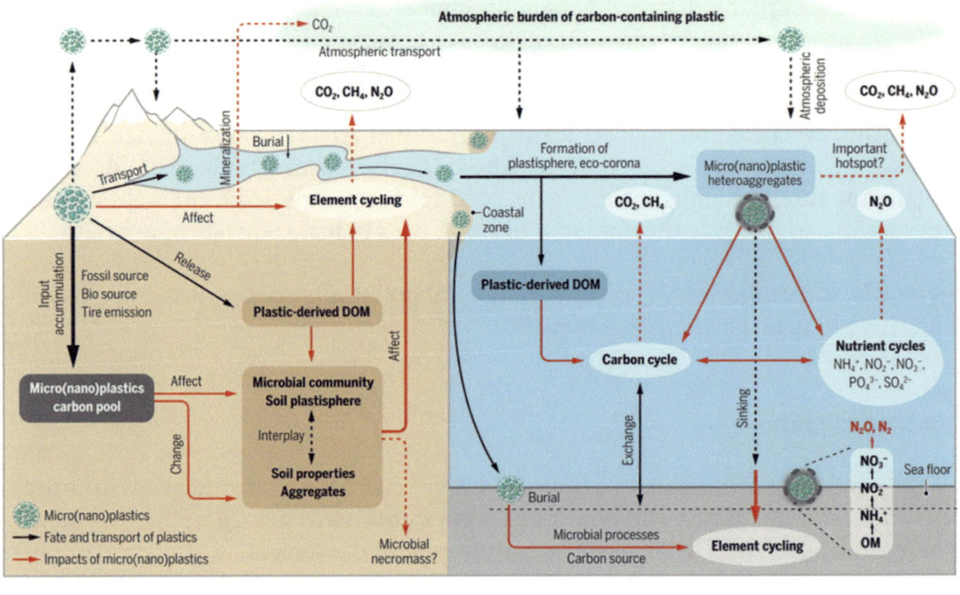

Figure 1.
MPs affect element biogeochemical cycles [9]. MP pollution is in the ocean, terrestrial ecosystem, fresh water, and atmosphere. MPs, plastic-derived dissolved organic matter, and the plastisphere can affect biogeochemical cycles of elements, including carbon, nitrogen, phosphorus, and sulfur; and fluxes of greenhouse gases through direct and indirect pathways. Determining the impact and extent of these processes requires additional observations and analysis. (© 2024 Science. All rights reserved.).

role in modulating biogeochemical cycles will be indispensable for comprehensively addressing the environmental implications of MP pollution.

Evidence of their potential imminent threat to human health continues to grow, as MPs have been increasingly detected in various consumables. Human exposure to MPs occurs through multiple pathways, including dietary intake (e.g., seafood, bottled water, milk, beer, and table salt), water consumption, and inhalation of air. It has since become increasingly recognized that the food chain is one of the key routes to human exposure to MPs, and that MPs have been identified in numerous food products. Moreover, the presence of MPs has been observed in a variety of human organ systems, such as the digestive, respiratory, circulatory, reproductive, nervous, immune, endocrine, urinary, and locomotor systems (**Figure 2**).

1.2 Human exposure pathways

Human exposure to MPs occurs predominantly through ingestion and inhalation. Dietary sources, including seafood, drinking water, and food packaged in plastic materials, contribute substantially to ingestion-based exposure. Additionally, airborne MPs, prevalent in both indoor and outdoor environments, represent a critical pathway through respiratory inhalation. This multifaceted exposure has raised significant public health concerns due to the potential systemic impacts of accumulated MPs within human tissues.

Exposure via ingestion is mostly linked to the intake of contaminated foodstuffs and beverages with dietary sources being major sources of these contaminants, which include seafood (mostly fish, bivalves, and crustaceans), drinking water (tap and bottled water), and foods packed or stored in plastic materials as the primary cause of ingestion-related exposures [10, 11]. High levels of MPs have been found in

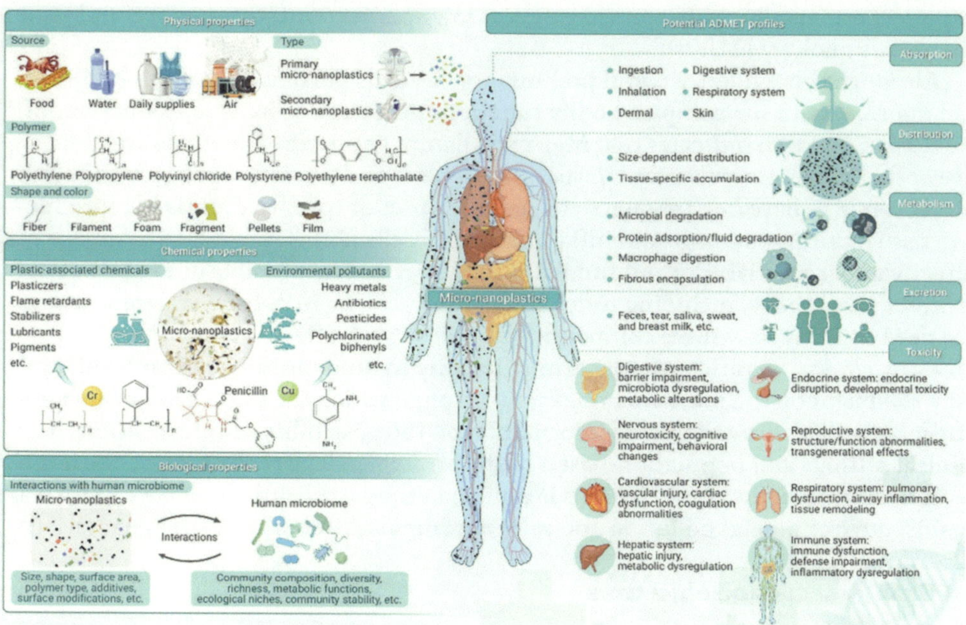

Figure 2.
The proposed comprehensive MP research framework. ADEMT: absorption, distribution, metabolism, excretion, and toxicity. (Copyright © 2025 Innovation Press).

many foods, such as sea salt, sugar, honey, milk products, processed foods, and most notably in seafood, as a result of rampant pollution of the sea [10, 12]. Drinking water is the second vital route of ingestion, and there is data evidence that bottled water, especially those in plastic bottles, is frequently more concentrated with MPs than tap water, as a result of the breaking off of particles of the bottles into which the water is filled and reused frequently [10, 13]. Also, MPs may be added to foods by plastic packaging and processing materials, which may release MPs during heating, storage conditions, and mechanical stress, contributing to the risk of dietary exposure [10, 12]. Babies and young children are potentially even more vulnerable; research has shown that the use of plastic feeding bottles and some food contact plastics could potentially liberate millions of MPs per day even under normal use conditions [10, 11]. The accumulation of MPs in human tissues is a relevant cause of metabolic disorders, immune changes, inflammation, and chronic diseases [14, 15].

Systemic consequences of MPs, particularly with chronic accumulation, can amount to an increased risk of gastrointestinal disorders, respiratory illnesses, cardiovascular diseases, metabolic syndrome, and even cancer owing to lingering inflammation and genome-damaging impacts [13, 16, 17]. Because of their widespread sources and the difficulty of eliminating them once inside the body, MPs pose a serious and burgeoning threat to global public health [18, 19].

1.3 Rationale for focusing on male reproductive health

Emergent data are increasingly indicating the harmful effects of MPs on biological systems, and specifically, there are concerns about the effects related to their impact on reproductive health [20]. A critical area of focus is the male reproductive system that is highly sensitive to environmental MPs. With increased environmental pollution around the globe, reduced male fertility has been observed and has been pointed to poor sperm quality indicators in terms of low sperm count, dysmotility, and poor sperm morphology [21].

Although this evidence is still preliminary, it yields persuasive signs that MPs can interfere with the complex bodily functions necessary to male reproduction. In particular, research indicates that MPs may disrupt endocrine functionality, thus disrupting hormone levels vital in spermatogenesis and general reproductive health. Moreover, MPs have been shown to trigger the onset of oxidative stress in reproductive tissue, causing damage and inflammation of cells [22]. The oxidative damage may directly affect the viability and functioning of sperm. The possible direct toxicity of reproductive organs, including testes and epididymis, by MPs further demonstrates the need to know how these compounds can cause such effects and whether they pose any clinical significance concerning fertility in humans. This research will not only shed light on the mechanisms exactly through which the MPs cause a damaging effect but will also give valuable information on the possibility of interventions in clinical settings and population-based health strategies. The realization of the level of reproductive toxicity caused by MPs is critical in the establishment of successful ways against environmental pollution and safeguarding male fertility to later generations.

1.4 Chapter scope and objectives

This chapter systematically reviews the current knowledge of how MPs impact male reproductive health, elucidating the biological mechanisms involved, such as oxidative stress induction, endocrine disruption, and structural damage to reproductive organs. Epidemiological findings that correlate MPs exposure with compromised male fertility parameters and increased infertility risks will be critically analyzed. Additionally, animal model studies will be examined to indicate dose-response relationships and potential transgenerational effects. Ultimately, this review aims to emphasize the urgency of advancing research and implementing targeted public health interventions to mitigate MPs' harmful reproductive consequences.

2. Environmental ubiquity and human exposure to MPs

2.1 Sources and formation of MPs

MPs originate from various anthropogenic sources, broadly classified into primary and secondary forms.

Primary MPs are deliberately manufactured particles for both consumer and industrial applications, including microbeads in personal care products and industrial abrasives. Owing to physical, chemical, and biological breakdown, secondary MPs turn to fragmentation and degradation of pieces of larger plastic waste. Such downstream breakage contributes to the increasing environmental load of MPs.

2.1.1 Primary MPs

Primary MPs are small plastic pieces under 5 mm. Their size ranges from 10 μm to 1 mm. Most pieces are spherical or cylindrical. They have smooth surfaces and uniform polymer composition. Recent studies report that polyethylene (PE) is the most common (42%), followed by polypropylene (PP, 28%); polyester is also prevalent [23]. These plastics originate from microbeads in personal care products, textile fibers, and pre-production plastic pellets. Personal care items and cosmetics, such as toothpaste, face wash, hand soap, and sunscreen, contain microbeads. The EU has banned microbeads in many of these products, yet manufacturers continue to use them because they are cost-effective and perform well.

MPs also accumulate in oral care materials. Researchers have detected polymethyl methacrylate and polyvinyl siloxane in toothpaste, toothbrush bristles, dental floss, and mouthwash [24]. A single use of an exfoliant or toothpaste can release between 4,500 and 95,500 microbeads [25]. Washing synthetic textiles releases fiber MPs; approximately 35% of these fibers enter wastewater [26].

Primary MPs are ubiquitous in aquatic and terrestrial environments. Fibers account for 49–70% of MPs in global wastewater and are primarily released during textile manufacturing and laundering [26]. Fiber shedding during washing constitutes 4–35% of all primary MPs emissions [5]. The expansion of the apparel industry exacerbates this pollution [27].

Beyond personal care products, industries produce MPs beads for numerous applications. They are used as plasticizers, fillers, and pigments in coatings and paints. These beads often carry additional chemical additives [28]. Another significant source is tire wear; abrasion generates persistent MPs particles that harm soil and aquatic microbial communities [29]. Studies also show that up to 84% of atmospheric MPs originate from road traffic, primarily tire wear.

2.1.2 Secondary MPs

Plastic items break down into secondary MPs in three ways (**Figure 3**), including UV light, physical abrasion, and biological ingestion. Microbes can attach and break down plastics into particles. MPs fibers make extra trouble. Textile fibers release many particles when washed or stretched [30].

Plastic use has grown fast around the world. Experts say it creates more waste than other pollutants. Poor waste control sends much plastic into the oceans. In 2010, oceans held 12.7 million tons of plastic. Experts expect a 10-fold increase in waste by 2025. Waves and UV light split ocean plastics into tiny bits. Fish and other animals eat these bits, and their digestion makes even smaller particles of plastics [31].

Wastewater plants collect MPs from homes and factories. They trap microbeads from personal care items and catch fibers from synthetic clothes. Plant machines cut plastics into smaller pieces. This process raises MPs levels in water and sludge.

2.2 Environmental distribution of MPs

MPs have achieved extensive global distribution, pervading diverse ecosystems. Aquatic environments, including oceans, rivers, lakes, and groundwater, serve as significant reservoirs for MPs, facilitated by hydrological transport processes. Terrestrial ecosystems accumulate MPs primarily through agricultural practices, waste disposal, and atmospheric deposition. MPs also circulate extensively within the atmosphere, dispersing widely as airborne particles and subsequently depositing across varied landscapes, including urban and remote areas.

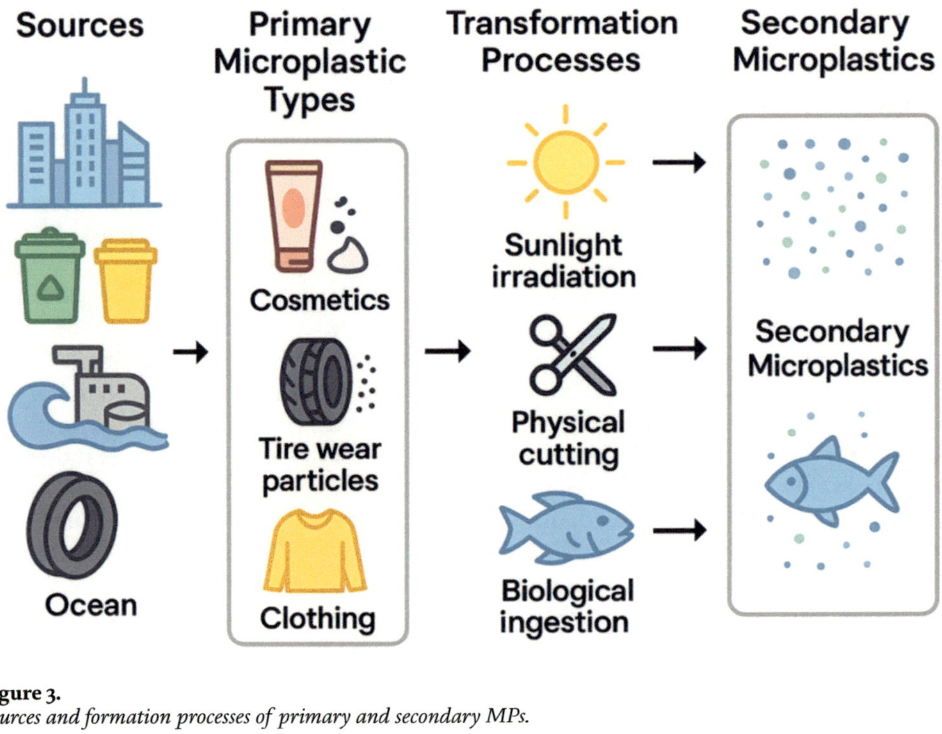

Figure 3.
Sources and formation processes of primary and secondary MPs.

2.3 Pathways of human exposure

2.3.1 Dietary intake (food and water)

The main sources of human dietary exposure to MPs are the consumption of tainted food and drinks. MPs have been reported widely in seafood, drinking water, and many packaged and processed food products (**Figure 2**). The ingestion pathway is particularly concerning due to the potential for MPs to accumulate in gastrointestinal tissues, leading to subsequent systemic distribution and physiological effects.

2.3.2 Inhalation of airborne particles

Inhalation represents another crucial route of human exposure to MPs, facilitated by indoor and outdoor air contaminated with suspended MP particles. These airborne MPs originate from textile fibers, vehicle tire abrasion, urban dust, and industrial emissions. Chronic inhalation exposure is associated with respiratory deposition and potential translocation to systemic circulation, raising health concerns about prolonged MP accumulation in pulmonary tissues.

2.4 Bio-accumulation in human tissues

Emerging evidence highlights the capability of MPs to bio-accumulate within human tissues, including the lungs, liver, intestines, and reproductive organs. Bio-accumulation occurs when exposure surpasses the body's elimination capacity, potentially leading to persistent biological effects. The accumulation of MPs in vital organs underscores the urgent need for comprehensive toxicological assessment and proactive public health strategies to mitigate exposure and adverse health outcomes.

2.4.1 Pathways of MP invasion and accumulation sites

Humans are exposed to MPs by ingestion, inhalation, and skin contact. Each person ingests 39,000 to 52,000 particles per year via food and drinking water [32]. These particles cross the gut lining, enter intestinal cells, move into the bloodstream, and build up in the gut and liver. People inhale about 272 MPs particles daily, and these particles can settle in the lungs and cause inflammation [33]. Many cosmetics and skincare products touch the skin, and particles under 100 nm can pass through the skin barrier and harm cell functions [34]. A study of tissue samples from individuals who died between 2016 and 2024 found MP concentrations of 4,917 μg/g in the brain, 433 μg/g in the liver, and 404 μg/g in the kidneys, with brain levels rising fastest [35]. MPs from food and water also travel to the reproductive system through the blood and can trigger inflammation and reduce sperm quality [36].

2.4.2 Mechanisms of MP bio-accumulation

Physicochemical properties drive MP accumulation in the human body. The body cannot clear these particles well. Small MP particles can cross tissue barriers. They move via lymphatic vessels and blood to tissues [37]. MPs surfaces are strongly hydrophobic. This trait lets them bind to cell membranes and plasma proteins. The binding can make them stay longer in tissues [38].

MPs also act as sponges for pollutants. They can adsorb heavy metals and organic toxins which boosts their bio-accumulation [39]. As a result, MPs often build up in almost all the organs in human body, such as the lungs, liver, kidneys, and reproductive organs (**Figure 4**) [40].

2.4.3 Potential health risks of MPs and public health implications

MP bio-accumulation is one of the serious health concerns, frequently causing endocrine disruption, oxidative stress, chronic inflammation, and tissue destruction [16]. It also found that MPs also can accumulate in the organs, such as the liver and kidneys. This buildup disrupts immune function. Researchers have indicated that the presence of MPs in the respiratory tract may lead to lung inflammation and breathing complications.

The reproductive system also suffers damage. MPs in reproductive organs cause pathological changes and lower germ-cell quality. This effect can harm offspring health. Nanoplastics can cross the blood-brain barrier. They induce oxidative stress and neuroinflammation. This action raises the risk of neurodegenerative diseases, such as Alzheimer's and Parkinson's [41].

MP pollution is widespread and long-lasting. Controlling MPs at its source is vital for public health. Authorities must set strict plastic-management standards. They

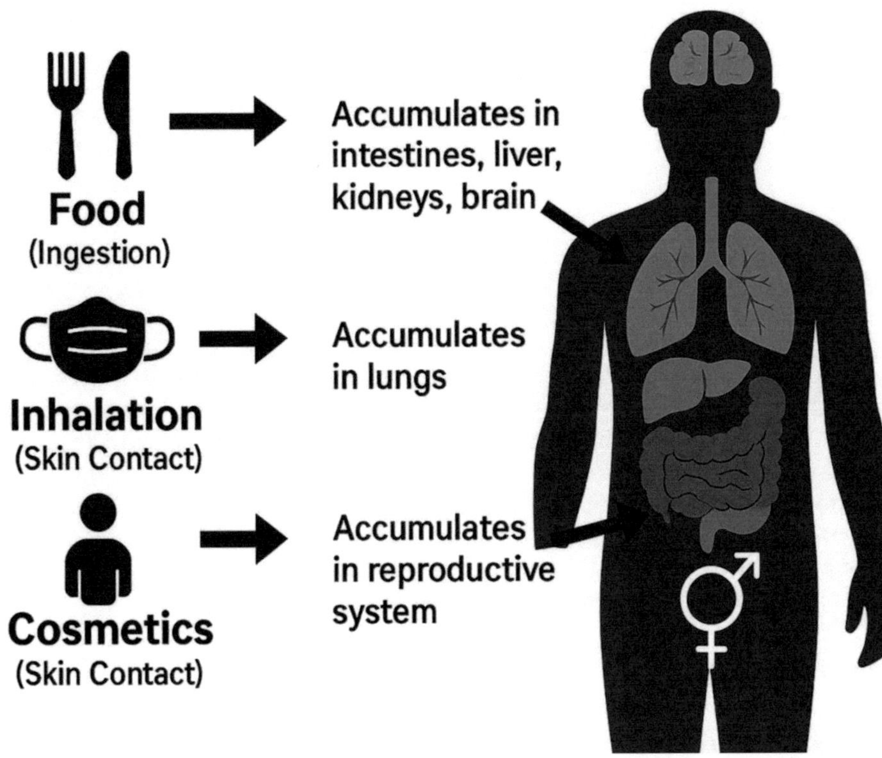

Figure 4.
MP pathways in the human body. By food, MPs can be accumulated in intestines, liver, kidneys, and the brain. By inhalation, MPs can be accumulated in the lung. By cosmetics (skin contact), MPs can be accumulated in the reproductive system.

must also define safe exposure limits. Research should expand epidemiological studies on human MP exposure. This work will clarify tissue-specific risks [42].

3. Adverse outcomes of MP exposure and mechanisms of MP-induced toxicity in male reproductive health

3.1 Adverse outcomes of MP exposure to male reproductive health

MP exposure negatively impacts male reproductive health through multiple mechanisms, including reduced testosterone level, spermatogenetic cells, luteinizing hormone, and follicle-stimulating hormone, as well as the induction of inflammatory responses and DNA damage (**Figure 5**). Principal adverse effects of MPs encompass several critical aspects: (a) reproductive dysfunction, presenting diversely and ultimately impairing overall reproductive capacity [44]; (b) parameter alterations in biochemical, spermatogenic, and histological aspects, indicative of disturbances within the sophisticated physiological processes essential for sperm production and male reproductive health [45]; (c) reductions in testosterone concentrations, a hormone critical for sustaining male reproductive functions and secondary sexual characteristics [46]; and (d) the initiation of oxidative stress and inflammatory pathways, triggering detrimental cascades that adversely affect sperm quality and testicular integrity [47]. Collectively, these adverse outcomes have profound implications for male reproductive fitness and fertility rates. Elucidating the underlying mechanisms linking MP exposure to these reproductive impairments is critical for developing targeted preventive arrangements and therapeutic interventions aimed at safeguarding and improving male reproductive health.

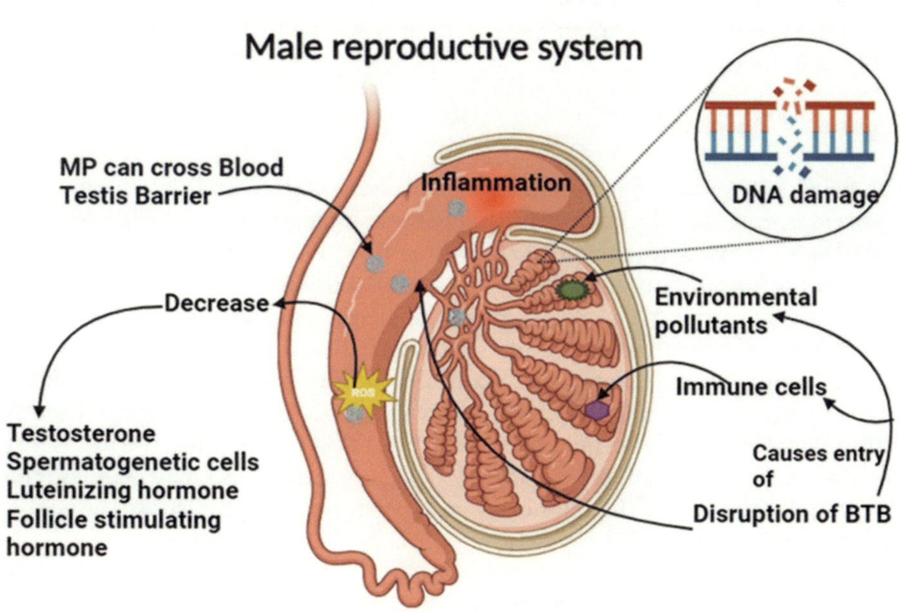

Figure 5.
MPs decrease testosterone, spermatogenetic cells, luteinizing hormone (LH), and follicle-stimulating hormone, causing inflammation and DNA damage [43]. (Copyright © 2025. Published by Springer Nature).

Emerging evidence elucidates a multi-factorial pathophysiology underlying MP-induced toxicity in the male reproductive system. The principal mechanisms involve oxidative stress and testicular injury, endocrine disruption, inflammatory responses, and potential dose-response and transgenerational effects. Together, these pathways disrupt the structural and functional integrity of male reproductive tissues and contribute to impaired fertility. It has been well-documented that MPs are harmful to male reproductive health due to the disruption of physiological and cellular procedures at several levels of the reproductive system, mainly through the mechanism associated with oxidative stress, endocrine disruption, immunotoxicity, and the intergenerational accumulation of the injuries [48, 49].

3.2 Oxidative stress and testicular injury

3.2.1 Generation of reactive oxygen species

Exposure to MPs has been shown to significantly elevate the generation of reactive oxygen species (ROS) within testicular tissue [50]. The resultant oxidative milieu overwhelms endogenous antioxidant defenses, promoting lipid peroxidation and cellular dysfunction. Oxidative stress has been linked to testicular damage and impaired Leydig cell function, which is crucial for testosterone synthesis.

The exposure of the tissues to MPs, especially polystyrene MPs (PS-MPs), causes an excessive generation of ROS in testicular tissues [51]. Abundant ROS overruns endogenous antioxidant defense system made up of enzymes/high activity that include superoxide dismutase (SOD), catalase, and glutathione peroxidase causing systemic and localized oxidative stress within testis [46]. These ROS, such as superoxide anion, hydrogen peroxide, and hydroxyl radicals, engage in lipid peroxidation, modify proteins, and disrupt mitochondrial functions, which can significantly compromise cellular homeostasis, both in somatic cells and germ cells [52]. This oxidative stress is dose-dependent and it escalates according to the proportion of MP concentration [53].

3.2.2 Sperm DNA damage

Enhanced ROS production facilitates DNA fragmentation and chromatin instability in spermatozoa, thereby compromising genetic integrity and reducing fertilization potential. Spermatozoa are exceptionally vulnerable to oxidative stress, due to their high concentrations of polyunsaturated fatty acids and low antioxidant potential [54]. Due to exposure to MPs, a ROS causes impairment of the nuclear DNA and mitochondrial DNA by attacking them, resulting in breaking the DNA, changing the bases, and forming cross-links of chromatin [55]. It is reflected in the DNA damage in the form of higher fragmentation index and formation of mutagenic lesions, including 8-hydroxy-2′-deoxyguanosine (8OHdG) that undermines the integrity of genetic material transferred to the oocyte [56]. The given effects may decrease the fertilization capacity, raise the rates of sperm apoptosis, and predispose the congenital disorders or infertility [53].

3.2.3 Disruption of the blood-testis barrier

MP exposure disrupts the BTB, as evidenced by altered expression of tight junction proteins and increased permeability. This disturbance renders germ cells vulnerable to toxic insults and immune-mediated damage. This special micro-environment is acquired by the BTB, composed mainly of tight junctions between adhering Sertoli cells, which help maintain a specialized micro-environment needed by spermatogenesis [57]. Oxidative stress generated by MPs, along with the activation of signal transduction cascades (carefully MAPK-Nrf2), results in the disruption of the nature of the BTB [58]. Experimental evidence indicates that the exposure to MPs leads to the down-regulation of the most significant proteins related to BTB (e.g., ZO-1, occludin), the rise of permeability, and the induction of apoptosis of germ cells in seminiferous tubules [59]. Immunological cells and toxic substances can destroy germ cells through BTB, leading to aberrant spermatogenesis and infertility [57, 60].

3.3 Endocrine disruption

3.3.1 Impaired hormonal regulation

MPs exert endocrine-disrupting effects by interfering with the hypothalamic-pituitary-gonadal (HPG) axis. Alterations in gonadotropin and androgen signaling have been observed following MP exposure [20, 61]. The HPG axis is significantly damaged by MPs through hormonal inhibition and oxidative stress, and testosterone deficiency is one of the key consequences [20]. Long-term exposures are also serious hazardous to male fertility among species, which requires more stringent environmental control and therapeutic intervention [61]. MPs interfere with the HPG axis either by interfering with or by imitating the endogenous hormones, thereby resulting in the alteration of the secretion pattern of main regulators. Prolonged exposure to MP, the hypothalamic gonadotropin-releasing hormone (GnRH) release is inhibited, and consequently, LH and follicle-stimulating hormone (FSH) synthesis in the pituitary are suppressed [62]. It was reported that PS-MPs (5 μm; 0.1 mg/L, 90 days) decreased serum LH (32%) and FSH (28%) in male mice compared with controls, with a direct impairment of Leydig cell functioning; and due to MP-induced oxidative stress, it causes testicular oxidative stress and peroxidation of testicular lipids, thereby lowering testosterone production by inhibiting steroidogenic enzymes (e.g., 17β-HSD). This interference occurs through receptor antagonism, as MPs take up estrogen/androgen receptors, thereby altering feedback loops [63]. This imbalance interferes with the regulation of the reproductive hormones, thereby reducing the hormonal support for normal testicular functioning and spermatogenesis [64].

3.3.2 Alteration of testosterone synthesis

Experimental data demonstrate significant reductions in intratesticular and circulating testosterone concentrations, attributable to the down-regulation of steroidogenic enzymes and Leydig cell dysfunction [65]. Long-term exposure of PS-MPs strongly inhibits LH receptor in Leydig cells. This inhibition disrupts the LHR/cAMP/PKA/steroidogenic acute regulatory (StAR) signal, which is the pathway to the production of testosterone in the body [61, 66]. The second important mechanism is the inhibition of the StAR protein, which transports cholesterol into mitochondria—a rate-limiting process in testosterone synthesis. In mouse models, PS-MPs have been demonstrated to decrease StAR expression by more than 50%, thus inhibiting the supply of testosterone precursors [61]. Besides this, MPs can also lead to oxidative stress by causing excessive production of ROS that promotes mitochondrial dysregulation. This involves exhaustion of antioxidant defense, including glutathione peroxidase 1 (GPX1). Depletion of GPX1 goes a step further to compound the effects of testosterone reduction about 40%, underscoring their protective effect from oxidative damage [67]. Bax/BCL-2 imbalance also stimulates apoptosis. The effects by MP exposure include up-regulation of pro-apoptotic protein Bax and down-regulation of anti-apoptotic protein BCL-2 [68]. The release of cytochrome C and activation of the caspase-3 eventually result in apoptosis of Leydig cells through this imbalance [69]. MPs also interfere with the GRP78/PERK/CHOP pathway. The activation of ER stress sensors (GRP78) by PS-MPs results in the phosphorylation of the PERK and up-regulation of CHOP. In its turn, CHOP facilitates apoptosis and inhibits the expression of such steroidogenic enzymes as CYP11A1 [70].

3.3.3 Effects on spermatogenesis

Disruption of hormonal homeostasis and direct toxicant action collectively impair spermatogenic processes, leading to decreased sperm production and maturation, and testosterone level may decrease by up to 57% [71]. MPs interfere with the hypothalamic-pituitary-testis axis and prevent the release of the pituitary LH and FSH, thus limiting the stimulation of spermatogenesis [72, 73]. The BTB may be breached by MPs and this is associated with the activation of oxidative stress and cellular damage. This causes an excess formation of ROS, fragmentation of the DNA, and impairment of the mitochondrial functioning in the germ cells, such as spermatogonia and spermatocytes [74, 75]. It has been recorded a 2.8-fold increase in the activity of caspase-3 in germ cells to which MPs/NPs were administered. Histological assessment reveals an extensive loss of spermatogonia (40%), spermatocytes (38%), and round spermatids (52%) [76]. Cadmium exposure model, analogous to MP metal carriers, as an analog of MP-related metals, showed an increased dose of spermatids. In addition, seminiferous tubules become smaller with a decrease in their diameter of 28–35% and epithelial thickening [74]. The tight junctions between Sertoli cells integrity are disturbed, and especially, claudin-11 keeps the integrity of the BTB. All of these harms occur to the sperm severely, including a 30–63% decline in total sperm count, a 41% diminishment in sperm in motion, and a 2.5-fold upsurge in morphological deformities. Exposure to MPs has also resulted in deformity of the sperm head and acrosomal loss [74]. The epididymal reserves of sperm decline by 58%, and fertilization *in vitro* by 72% in the MP-treated models [74].

3.4 Inflammatory responses and immunotoxicity

MPs induce local and systemic inflammatory responses, characterized by up-regulation of pro-inflammatory cytokines and infiltration of immune cells into testicular tissue. Chronic inflammation contributes to further oxidative damage and exacerbates reproductive toxicity. Pattern recognition receptors such as TLR4 and NLRP3 inflammasomes in testicular macrophages and Sertoli cells are stimulated by MPs [77]. This promotes the processes of NF-κB and MAPK that increases pro-inflammatory cytokines TNF-α, IL-1β, and IL-6 in the testicular tissue [78]. TNF-α accelerates inflammation through the formation of ROS, whereas IL-1β attracts neutrophils and macrophages [79, 80]. Inflammatory downregulation of tight junction proteins (claudin-5, occludin, ZO-1) occurs through ERK phosphorylation mediated through TNF-α [81]. Loss of BTB integrity allows infiltration of immune cells and penetration of antibodies such that the germ cells are vulnerable to an autoimmune attack [75]. Cytokine storms trigger the dysfunction of mitochondrial functions and the apoptotic program (by activating caspase-3/9) in an ROS-dependent manner. TNF-α also inhibits steroid oil enzymes (STAR, CYP11A1) to lower the testosterone biosynthesis, which is vital in spermatogenesis; and in other avian models, PS-MPs modeled BTB destruction and thickening of the basement membrane, which is directly proportional to poor sperm quality [75]. Inflammation of other organs mediated by cytokine spill over into circulation is initiated by MPs. Tests on spleen immunotoxicity indicate experimentally that microglia-like reactions triggered by MP increase systemic TNF-α/IL-1β production by several folds [82, 83]. Repeated exposure can disrupt testicular immune privilege because it exposes the apoptotic testicular germ cells with neo-antigens that in turn trigger the production of anti-sperm antibodies as shown in **Table 1** [81].

3.5 Dose-response and transgenerational effects

Animal model studies reveal a dose-dependent relationship between MP exposure and reproductive impairment, with chronic low-dose exposure sufficient to induce subclinical pathology. Notably, preliminary evidence suggests the possibility of transgenerational effects, as epigenetic alterations and impaired reproductive outcomes have been documented in offspring of exposed animals [84]. MP exposure caused testicular damage in a dose-dependent mechanism that is largely caused by oxidative stress, apoptosis, and hormone deficiency [85]. In mice that received chronic exposure to PS-MPs (MPs; 0.25–1 mg/kg/d) by 4–21 w, sperm concentration and mobility decreased by 36% and 15.7%, respectively [46, 86]. As low as 2 μg/L MPs reportedly stimulated seminiferous tubule deterioration and Leydig cell atrophy. The level of antioxidant enzymes (e.g., catalase, SOD) dropped by 40–50% at the concentration of 200 μg/L [84]. The inhibitory effect of MPs on the expression of LHR leads to a 33.3% reduction in the production of testosterone through disruption of the LHR/cAMP/PKA/StAR pathway in the hormonal axis [87]. By ROS-mediated apoptotic cascades, MPs stimulate NOX4/NF-kB signaling, inducing mitochondrial apoptosis (caspase-3 ↑200%) in spermatogonia in a dose-dependent manner. Similarly, PS-MPs castrate androgen receptor expression [88] by 60%, and spermiation is inhibited in a dose-dependent manner [86, 89]. The accumulation of damage caused by MP is progressively associated with transgenerational inheritance through epigenetic transmission in the germline. Indeed, some of the previous studies have indicated that sperm DNA methylation patterns are highly changed in the offspring of PS-MP-exposed mice [90, 91]. Hypermethylation, in particular, of genes related to spermatogenesis (including *StAR* and *Akr1c1*) led to a loss of fertility by 25–30% in both F1 and F2 generation. Regarding histone modifications, *Caenorhabditis elegans* exposure to the amino-modified PS nanoparticles in the parental generation (100 μg/L) resulted

Pathway	Key effector	Reproductive impact
ROS/NF-κB axis	TNF-α ↑, IL-1β ↑, COX2 ↑	BTB rupture, steroidogenesis ↓
MAPK activation	p38/JNK phosphorylation	Germ cell apoptosis
Lysosomal damage	Cathepsin B release	NLRP3 inflammasome activation
Autoantibody generation	Anti-sperm IgG production	Immune-mediated infertility

Table 1.
Inflammatory responses via MP exposure in testis.

in the 3.5-fold up-regulation of the repressive histone mark H3K27me3 [90, 91]. This was an epigenetic alteration that led to ovarian immaturity in the offspring of unexposed F3 generations, as one means of multi-generation effect [90, 91]. They have also characterized the dysregulation of non-coding RNA, where F1 mouse sperm has shown up-regulation of miR-34c and miR-449a, both associated with high apoptosis and sperm maturation dysregulation [92, 93]. The overall evidence indicates that exposure to MPs may trigger heritable epigenetic change with long-lasting effects on reproduction [94].

In summary, MPs compromise male reproductive health through a convergence of oxidative stress, DNA and tissue injury, hormonal dysregulation, inflammation, and possible heritable effects. These observations indicate the necessity to conduct further research to fully understand the mechanisms of MP exposure and the long-term effects.

Empirical Evidence Linking MPs to Male Reproductive Impairment.

3.6 Epidemiological findings

The effects of MP exposure on male reproduction are under the early stages of epidemiological studies; however, they are rapidly gaining attention due to the alarming ubiquity of MPs in the environment. Despite a lack of direct evidence pointing to the negative impact that MP contamination has on human reproductive health, the impact of environmental pollution, particularly, the presence of particulate matter, has been studied extensively with regard to its deleterious impact on human health [95, 96].

This evidence supports and emphasizes upgrading the necessity to deeply investigate all the possible sources that lead to a decline in male reproductive health with the possible involvement of MPs.

3.6.1 The association between plastic production and male reproductive health

The global surge in plastic production, notably driven by China's industrial expansion over the past five decades (1970s–2020s), has coincided markedly with a pronounced deterioration in the semen quality among donors, with an especially steep decline observed from 2010 onward (**Figure 6**) [97, 98]. This observation underscores a troubling inverse correlation, wherein the expansion of the plastic industry parallels a significant regression in male reproductive health. Concurrently, the extensive use and disposal of plastic products in these 50 years have led to extensive environmental contamination, characterized by the breakdown of plastic into MPs. These MPs have been demonstrated to infiltrate various biological pathways within the human body, including penetration of the blood-testis barrier and subsequent accumulation within the reproductive tissues [97, 98].

This infiltration of MPs into reproductive organs poses substantial risks to human fertility and raises critical concerns regarding the health of future generations. Furthermore, declining birth rates observed in major global economies are contributing to demographic shifts toward population aging, a phenomenon with profound and wide-ranging implications. Consequently, the nexus between plastic pollution and declining reproductive health constitutes not merely an urgent public health issue but also a socioeconomic challenge with extensive global repercussions.

Several population-based studies have provided insights into the association between MP exposure and reduced sperm quality [99, 100]. Lower sperm count,

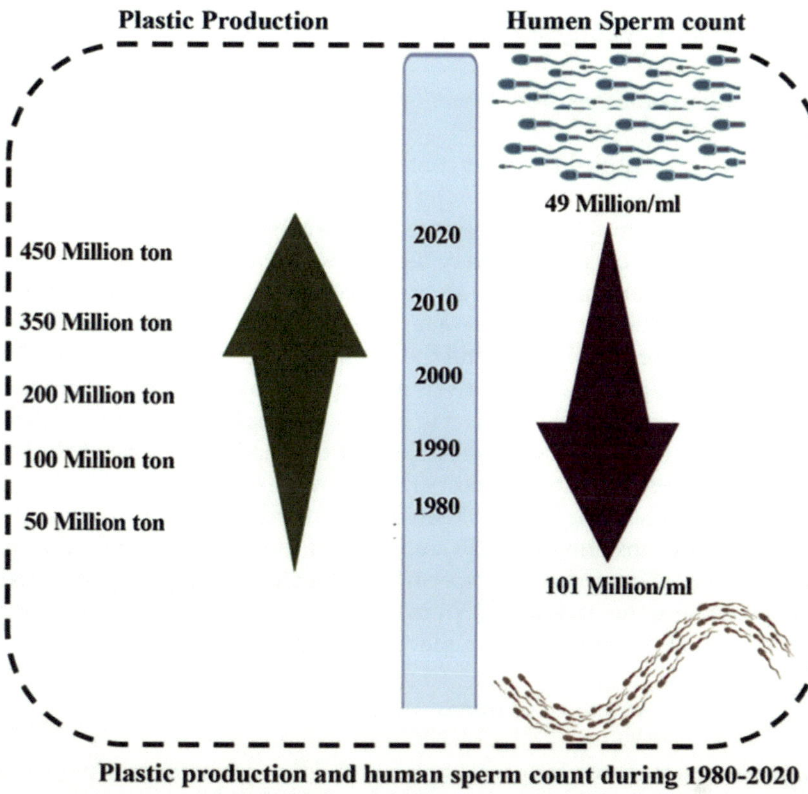

Figure 6.
Trends in plastic yield and semen quality of donors in the 1970s–2020s.

morphology, and motility have consistently been reported in male residing in regions with high environmental contamination of MPs. The environmental PS or PE, with sizes ranging from 20 nm to 10 μm, and exposure doses ranging from 0.1 to 20 mg/L, have durations varying from 0.5 h to 35 d. Both *in vivo* and *in vitro* findings have provided evidences that MP can cause lower levels of testosterone and impair the BTB, testicular inflammation, and abnormality of spermatogenesis at the tissue and organ levels. All these have an impact of reducing the number and quality of sperm, and this is a major risk to male reproductive health [99]. These evidences imply that the degree of MP exposure, whether through contaminated food, water, or air, correlates with diminished semen quality.

Although the epidemiological evidence provides compelling data, there are notable limitations. Most studies are observational and suffer from confounding factors, such as lifestyle choices, occupational exposures, and underlying health conditions, which may also contribute to reproductive dysfunction. Future studies should prioritize detailed characterization of exposure thresholds, long-term reproductive sequelae, and elucidation of underlying molecular mechanisms to inform effective regulatory measures and mitigate the public health impact of MPs.

Furthermore, exposure assessment methodologies—often relying on indirect measures or self-reported data—limit the ability to accurately quantify MP exposure levels. Despite these challenges, the consistent findings across different populations and geographic regions underscore the need for more robust and controlled studies to confirm these associations and elucidate the underlying mechanisms.

3.6.2 Sperm quality parameters (count, motility, and morphology) and MP exposure

There is growing scientific literatures confirming the association between MP exposure and abnormal sperm parameters among humans [101]. Cross-sectional study noted a decrease in sperm concentration and sperm count in MP-exposed men, and data were showing 1.15×10^6/mL decrease with every IQR increase in $PM_{2.5}$ constituents (*e.g.*, black carbon, sulfate) [102]. Exposure to MPs also reduces progressive motility as it was found that PS-MPs was present in 85% of the semen samples, and there was a 30% decrease in motility with an increased MP burden and the loss of motility by the actions of p38 MAPK signaling and ROS [100]. MPs also negatively alter sperm motility and ATP production which are reflective of metabolic disorders in human studies (*e.g.*, VCL, VSL) [103]. Abnormal sperm morphology, such as the defects of the head and coiling of the tail, is related to MPs. The presence of teratozoospermia in men exposed to MPs increased by 1.8 times [100]. At the mechanistic level, polyamide MPs disrupt hormone balance, decrease the bioavailability of testosterone by 42%, and suppress the process of spermiogenesis [100]. The damages on the structure of sperm are also evident. It indicates the loss of acrosome and increased fragmentation of DNA in MP-exposed sperm, further confirming that MPs threaten male fertility on various levels [104, 105].

3.6.3 Male infertility prevalence and trends

The observed deterioration in sperm quality coincides with increasing prevalence rates of idiopathic male infertility in regions with substantial MPs contamination. Temporal analyses indicate a parallel trend between the escalation of environmental MP pollution and the global rise in male infertility rates, further substantiating a potential causal link. However, 7–10% of male population is affected by male infertility that comprises 40–50% of couple infertility cases and of which ~30–50 cases remain idiopathic [106, 107]. In the past decades, sperm quality has been adversely affected due to a ~ 16.4% decrease in sperm count and degraded motility and morphology [75]. This coincides with an increased exposure to MP pollutants. MPs disrupt the male reproductive system through oxidative stress, mitochondrial dysfunction, and endocrine disruption, and lower antioxidant defenses (*e.g.* SOD and CAT), ATP generation, and testosterone production [108]. NPs disintegrate BTB, encompass inflammation, and cause the loss of germ cells [109]. The epidemiological data demonstrate that high MP biomarkers are associated with 2- to 3-fold increased oligo- and asthenozoospermia risks in males [75]. It has been established that animal models validate MP-mediated testicular injury and adverse changes to spermatogenesis. In 83% of tap and 90% of bottled waters [75], particularly in industrial regions, a 15–20% increase in idiopathic male infertility has been reported in contaminated areas [110–112].

While epidemiological evidence strongly supports a correlation between MPs exposure and adverse male reproductive outcomes, further studies are essential to establish definitive dose-response relationships and to evaluate the long-term effects of such exposure. These findings call for immediate attention to the potential public health risks posed by MPs, urging both improved environmental policies and focused research efforts to mitigate their impact on human health.

Importantly, epidemiological studies for investigating the reproductive toxicity of MPs require adequately addressing and controlling potential confounding factors. Lifestyle choices such as dietary patterns, smoking, alcohol consumption, and physical activity levels, along with simultaneous exposure to other environmental contaminants (e.g., heavy metals, endocrine-disrupting chemicals), represent significant confounders capable of independently affecting male reproductive health. The careful consideration and adjustment for these variables in epidemiological analyses are imperative to accurately discern the specific contribution of MP exposure to reproductive outcomes.

Future studies should prioritize detailed investigations of exposure thresholds, the elucidation of molecular mechanisms underpinning toxicity, and comprehensive control for confounding lifestyle and environmental factors. Such rigorous approaches are essential to accurately inform regulatory policies and mitigate the public health risks associated with MP pollution.

3.7 Evidence from animal models

The animal experimentation has also played a pivotal role in explaining the mechanistic effects of exposure to MPs in male infertility, especially due to interruption of spermatogenesis as shown in **Table 2** [21]. The essential inferences on controlled experiments show dose-dependent spermatogenic dysfunction that can be

Species/model	Particle type/size	Exposure route and duration	Key spermatogenesis anomalies	Reference
Balb/c mice [113]	PS-MPs (1 μm), PS-NPs (70 nm)	Intratracheal instillation, 28 d	↑ Drp1/Fis1 (fission), ↓ Mfn1/Opa1 (fusion); ↓ sperm motility (34%); abnormal acrosomes	[113]
C57BL/6 mice [114]	PS-NPs (100 nm)	Oral gavage, 12 w	↓ Spermatogonia (27%); ↑ ROS; gut microbiota dysbiosis linked to spermatogenic arrest	[114]
ICR mice [115]	PS-MPs (5 μm), PS-NPs (50 nm)	Intraperitoneal, 12 w	↓ Sperm count (45%); ↑ sperm malformations; BTB disruption; ↓ Sertoli cell viability (30%)	[115]
Earthworms (*E. Andrei*) [116]	PE-MPs (10–200 μm)	Soil, 14 d	Fragmented NPs in testes; ↑ spermatocyte apoptosis; ↓ sperm bundle formation	[116]
Kunming mice [101]	PS-NPs (80 nm), PS-MPs (0.5 μm)	Oral, 8 weeks	↓ Testosterone (58%); ↓ spermatid count; ↑ caspase-3 (apoptosis); altered cAMP/PKA signaling	[101]
Sprague-Dawley rats [117]	PS-NPs (100 nm)	Oral, 10 w	↑ 8-OHdG (DNA damage); ↓ sperm viability; Leydig cell degeneration; IL-1β/TNF-α inflammation	[117]
CD-1 mice [118]	PS-NPs (25 nm)	Intravenous, 4 w	Transgenerational: ↓ F1 sperm quality; ↑ histone H3K27me3 in sperm	[118]

Table 2.
Summary of in vivo *microplastic exposure studies across major animal models and associated pathological effects.*

described as a potentiation of mitochondrial dysfunction, oxidative stress, endocrine disturbances, and epigenetic modifications.

Controlled animal experiments have provided critical insights into the reproductive toxicity of MPs. Rodent models, in particular, have enabled systematic examination of dose-response relationships by administering defined concentrations of MPs via ingestion or inhalation [46]. It suggested that dose- and size-specific toxicities exist, where smaller particles (0.08–0.5 μm) are more effective in penetrating the BTB and result in toxicity through oxidative stress [46]. It is quite interesting to point out that in circumstances where MPs have been co-exposed to phthalates or even when there were high-fat diets, synergistic reproductive toxicity has been observed [119]. The above studies have emphasized collectively about the role of particle size, exposure time, and environmental complexity in modifying reproductive outcomes.

Non-linear and typically non-monotonic toxicity patterns can be observed based on dose-response relationship. Although exposure to low-level PS-MPs can impair subcellular functions without causing gross tissue alterations, exposure to higher doses of PS-MPs can lead to oxidative stress, abrogation of the BTB, and apoptosis of germ cells [84]. Interestingly, hormonal disruptions have also been reported to be more significant at moderate doses (e.g. testosterone suppression at 5 mg/L greater than at 50 mg/L) and may be indicative of an endocrine-level compensatory effect. Quantitative risk assessment based on generalized linear models and Benchmark dose (BMD) modeling provides a framework to display sensitivity thresholds of reproductive toxicity recognizing BMD10 values, e.g., dose causing 10% effect for PS-MP-induced sperm count reductions in rats at 18.7 μg/kg/d [120]. Nonetheless, aspects like co-exposures matrices, species-specific sensitivity, and biodistribution kinetics complicate the equation and require a delicate toxicokinetic-toxicodynamic model that can adequately describe MP-related reproductive hazards [121].

3.8 Molecular biomarkers and mechanistic insights

Histopathological evaluation of reproductive tissues from exposed animals has revealed pronounced disruptions of the seminiferous epithelium, degeneration of spermatogenic cells, and thickening of the basement membrane [89]. Biochemical analyses further indicate increased levels of lipid peroxidation, decreased antioxidant enzyme activities, and elevated markers of DNA damage within testicular tissue [122]. These strategies demonstrate that treatments with MP exposure downregulate critical genes and signaling pathways implicated in testosterone biosynthesis, in particular, by inhibiting the LH-stimulated LHR/cAMP/PKA/StAR axis [46]. This interruption causes low testosterone production thus affecting spermatogenesis and sperm maturation. Up-regulation of stress, inflammation, and apoptotic pathways in testicular cells has also been observed in the multi-omics studies. Combining transcriptomics and metabolomics data yields a more complete diagram of the toxicity caused by MPs and contributes to the identification of early molecular biomarkers to be used as diagnostic and therapeutic targets [123]. Such biomarkers make it possible to monitor reproductive health on a minimally invasive basis and could inform clinical decisions in a timely manner.

Collectively, these outcomes substantiate the role of MPs in inducing oxidative stress and impairing the structural and functional integrity of the male reproductive system [67].

4. Research methodologies and knowledge gaps

The search to understand the connection between MP pollution and male health reproductive processes requires the unification of technical innovations and methodological approaches. These include:

a. Conducting environmental monitoring to accurately quantify MP concentrations and establish precise dose-response relationships. This surveillance aims to systematically evaluate the prevalence and toxicological impacts of MPs within specific environmental contexts and defined temporal periods.

b. Performing comprehensive analysis through systematic toxicology is combined with integrated multi-omics techniques. Such methods include differential gene expression analysis, differential protein expression profiling, and assessment of differential metabolite abundance. These methodologies encompass an assessment of semen quality, analysis of the integrity of BTB, measurement of MPs in semen, determination of biomarkers of biological damage, and characterization of multi-omics changes. Furthermore, establishing standardized protocols and robust analytical frameworks for MP detection and quantification in biological samples is imperative.

c. Investigating toxicological effects using both *in vivo* and *in vitro* studies in male animal models [124], which can provide critical insights and corroborating evidence regarding the health implications of MPs on the human male reproductive systems.

d. Identifying specific biomarkers [125], including proteins, DNA [126], RNA, and small molecular metabolites, as indicators of adverse effects on male reproductive health.

e. Synthesizing evidence from epidemiological investigations and conducting prospective, multi-center observational cohort studies.

These multidisciplinary methodologies are essential for advancing scientific understanding, addressing current knowledge gaps, and informing public health strategies aimed at mitigating the adverse effects of MPs on human reproductive health and the environmental safety.

4.1 Analytical techniques for MP detection

4.1.1 Environmental monitoring

Accurate environmental monitoring of MPs relies on sophisticated analytical techniques, such as Fourier-transform infrared spectroscopy (FTIR), Raman spectroscopy, and mass spectrometry-based methods [127]. These technologies facilitate precise identification, quantification, and characterization of MPs in diverse environmental matrices, essential for assessing ecological exposure levels and informing regulatory frameworks. **Table 3** illustrated the methodologies for detecting MPs.

Technique	Principle	Strengths	Limitations	Applications	References
Histological examination	Tissue sectioning and staining for MP visualization	*In situ* localization; assessment of tissue inflammation/toxicity	Low specificity for polymer identification; manual quantification bias	MP accumulation in testes, liver, and placenta; spermatogenesis disruption analysis	[114, 116, 125, 128]
Microscopy-spectroscopy Coupling	SEM/TEM imaging + μ-FTIR/μ-Raman	Morphological + chemical characterization; high-resolution NP detection	Sample dehydration artifacts; complex protocol standardization	MPs/NPs uptake in cellular/ subcellular structures; reproductive tissue analysis	[129–134]
Bioanalytical sensors	Surface-enhanced Raman scattering (SERS) or fluorescence tagging.	High sensitivity for NPs; real-time detection in biofluids.	Limited multiplexing; matrix interference in clinical samples; requires particle labeling.	Human blood/urine analysis; real-time NP detection in *Caenorhabditis elegans* models.	[135–138]
Chemometric profiling	Spectral data analysis deep learning).	Untargeted detection of biochemical alterations; high-throughput data integration.	Computational complexity; limited validation in human tissues.	HepG2 cell toxicity screening; spermatogenic cell damage assessment.	[139–142]

Table 3.
Summary of methodologies for detecting MPs.

4.1.2 Biological sample analysis

In biological systems, MP detection necessitates specialized methods, including histological examination, microscopy techniques coupled with spectroscopic confirmation, and advanced bioanalytical approaches [143]. These methodologies enable reliable assessment of MP bio-accumulation, distribution, and potential biological effects within human tissues, providing crucial data for risk assessment and health impact studies [144].

Semen analysis constitutes an essential component in the comprehensive assessment of infertility [145], offering valuable insights into male reproductive health. It has been established that plenty of factors may culminate in the observed challenge in male fertility; and this includes the probable effects of possible MPs on the reproductive system. The correlation between MPs exposure and male infertility cannot be overlooked [13]. Although direct causal evidence remains elusive, compelling evidence supports the proposition that chronic exposure to toxic effects of MPs may represent a significant risk factor for male reproductive dysfunction.

4.2 Advances in multi-omics and toxicological assessment

Recent advancements in multi-omics technologies, including genomics, proteomics, metabolomics, and transcriptomics, have significantly enriched our understanding of MP-induced toxicity.

4.2.1 Genomics epigenomics

MPs to spermatogenic cells trigger oxidative stress resulting in the impairment of genomic stability and DNA damage. This affects the process of meiosis and sperm maturation, leading to oligospermia or azoospermia [146, 147]. Transgenerational risks of infertility have been linked to epigenetic perturbations, including ectopic DNA methylation in critical genes related to the spermatogenesis process, including the HOX and FOX genes [148].

4.2.2 Transcriptomics

It has been shown that MP exposure can change the expression of genes essential in spermatogenesis (e.g., TEX101, PRM1), mainly by disrupting the process of hormone production, such as testosterone biosynthesis. Also, there are up-regulated non-coding RNAs like miR-34a, which impedes the activity of Sertoli cells and decreases the motility of sperm [149].

4.2.3 Proteomics metabolomics

The proteomic seminal plasma analysis indicates the down-regulation of the sperm adhesion proteins (e.g., ACRBP, ZPBP), and the up-regulation of immune activation components (e.g., IL-6, TNF-a), indicating the immune activation and sperm-egg binding failure [150].

4.2.4 Metabolomic analysis

It reveals impaired ATP synthesis and maladaptation of lipid metabolism, which degrades the motility of sperms [128]. Moreover, depletion of antioxidants causes the accumulation of lipid peroxides that include malondialdehyde, which further enhances oxidative damage [147].

These comprehensive analytical platforms elucidate molecular alterations and pathways activated by MPs exposure, offering insights into the mechanistic basis of reproductive impairment and enabling identification of novel biomarkers and therapeutic targets.

4.3 Testicular organoids (TOs): A cutting-edge platform for MP toxicology research

TOs represent an optimal *in vitro* model to perform MP-mediated testicular toxicity studies, which can deliver truly physiologically relevant data that fall between the two extremes of traditional cell cultures and *in vivo* models shown in **Table 4**. The 3D structures self-assemble to recapitulate the native testis architecture, into which they integrate major cell types, including Sertoli cells, Leydig cells, peritubular myoid cells, and germ cells, to create compartmentalized, tubule-like structures [129]. Their functional support of testosterone hormone-responsive release includes germ cell maturation to early spermatids, at least in murine models [130]. Notably, the TO platform also recapitulates the BTB and serves as an excellent model to evaluate the disruptive properties of MPs regarding the localization of germ cells and the immune privilege of the testis [131]. Their applicability runs toward high throughput toxicity screening with the potential to analyze quantitatively MP-associated oxidative stress, apoptosis, impaired spermatogenesis, and endocrine disruption. ATP-based viability stress tests, caspase activation, spermatid depletions, and losses of testosterone production, up to 40–60% in exposed murine organoids can also be used to measure these endpoints [135].

In addition to the assessment of phenotype, TOs have the potential to contribute mechanistic details of MP toxicity by uptake studies and multi-omics profiling (**Figure 7**). The uptake of MPs by Sertoli cells through endocytosis and their accumulation promote the activation of inflammatory pathways mediated by NF-kB and radically disrupt testicular homeostasis [136]. Transcriptomics and proteomics also demonstrate abnormal expression of several significant genes and pathways, including a down-regulation of the *CYP17A1* gene, which plays an important role in testosterone biosynthesis [139]. They can also be used to assess their therapeutic interventions, with antioxidants, such as *Ginkgo biloba* extract, having the potential to decrease apoptosis by a factor of up to 50 through SKP2 induction [140], and nanomaterial-based scavengers of MPs having an efficacy of up to 70% in reducing cytotoxicity. Combinations of organoid technology with state-of-the-art bio-materials and omics technologies will enable the researchers to discover the molecular mechanisms of MP toxicity and protective strategies. With further advancements,

Parameter	Animal models	2D cultures	TOs
Physiological relevance	Moderate	Low	High [129, 151]
Throughput	Low	Moderate	High [151, 152]
Human translatability	Limited	Limited	High [153, 154]
Multi-omics compatibility	Complex	Feasible	Optimal [155, 156]

Table 4.
The advantages of organoids over conventional models.

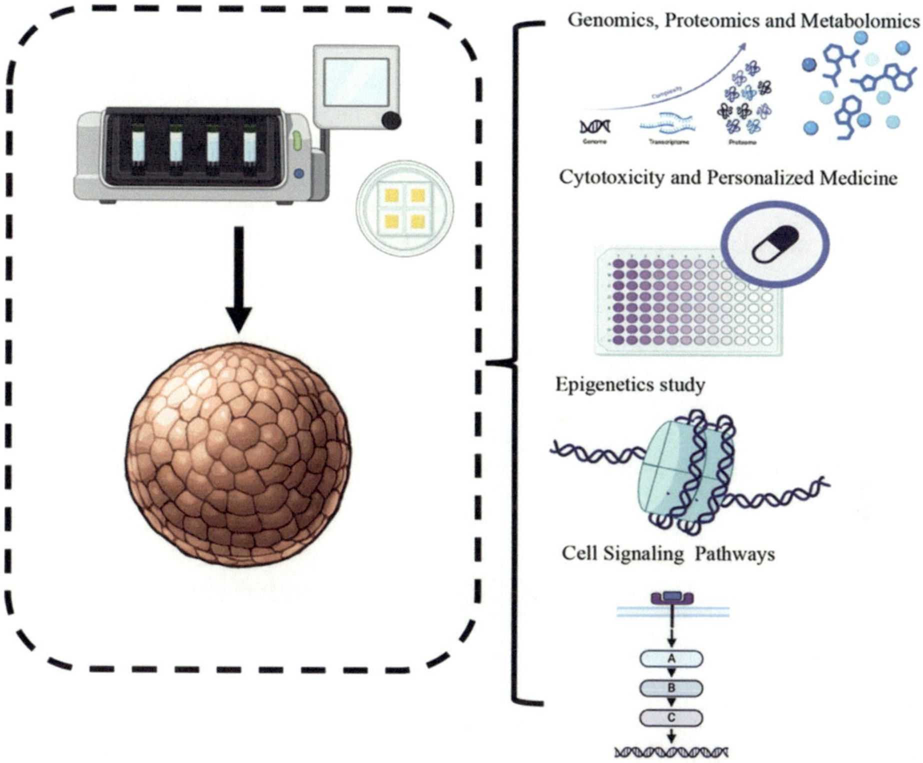

Figure 7.
The working principle and research strategy of TOs. The integrative strategy for testing MP toxicity with TOs. Genomics, proteomics, and metabolomics can be used to determine the molecular changes caused by MPs, including the measurements of cell viability/activity, and facilitate risk analysis of specific reproductive diseases. It can be also used for the examination of the effects on hereditary modifications (e.g., methylating DNA) of exposure to MP and decoding the MP-stimulated cascades (e.g., oxidative stress, steroidogenesis).

especially in vascularization and full support of spermatogenesis, TOs will be an inevitable subject with reproductive toxicology and environmental health studies [157].

4.4 Challenges in establishing causality

Despite considerable progress, establishing definitive causal links between MP exposure and adverse reproductive outcomes remains challenging due to complexities in exposure assessment, variability in human susceptibility, and concurrent exposure to multiple environmental contaminants. Addressing these issues requires rigorous epidemiological designs, controlled experimental studies, and integration of robust exposure assessment methodologies.

MP exposure and its assessment are complex. MPs can be absorbed through diet, inhalation, and skin contact. They can be present in varying concentrations and types in different environments. This variation poses a big challenge to MP monitoring [158]. The sample preparation of MPs has not been standardized, and the detection limits of MP detection methods are undefined [159]. Most people face long-term low-dose MP exposure. Scientists must clarify the dose response at these levels. This step is a key for realistic health risk assessment [160].

Age, sex, lifestyle, and job type shape how people react to MPs. The same exposure can cause different health effects. One study tested 2,000 adults and found that MP levels in saliva, skin, and hair vary by sex, ethnicity, and living conditions [161]. They often clump into aggregates and attract organic pollutants, heavy metals, and pathogens. That means MPs also can be acted as carriers. This mix boosts the toxicity of plasticizers, metals, and drug-resistant bacteria [161]. This co-contamination raises health risks.

4.5 Need for standardization and longitudinal studies

Standardized protocols for MP detection, quantification, and toxicity evaluation are critically needed to facilitate comparability across studies and improve the reliability of findings. Furthermore, longitudinal cohort studies are imperative to assess chronic exposure effects, temporal trends, and potential transgenerational implications. Advancing research through standardized and longitudinal methodologies will significantly enhance the precision of risk assessment and inform evidence-based public health interventions.

5. Public health implications and policy recommendations

5.1 Socioeconomic and demographic impacts

The pervasive exposure to MPs represents a significant and growing public health concern with disproportionate effects across socioeconomic and demographic strata. Populations residing in regions with inadequate waste management infrastructure, lower socioeconomic status, and limited access to health education are at increased risk of MP exposure. Such disparities may compound preexisting health inequalities, particularly concerning male reproductive health outcomes. Demographic variables, including age, occupational exposure, and dietary habits, further modulate individual susceptibility. Addressing these inequities requires comprehensive policy measures that prioritize vulnerable populations and integrate social determinants of health into MP exposure mitigation strategies.

5.2 Strategies for exposure mitigation

5.2.1 Source reduction and regulation

Effective reduction of human MP exposure necessitates coordinated regulatory interventions at both national and international levels. Source reduction should prioritize the restriction of primary MPs in consumer products and industrial applications, coupled with stringent regulation of plastic waste management and recycling processes. The implementation of robust environmental standards and enforcement mechanisms is essential to curtail the release of MPs into the ecosystem. Additionally, fostering innovation in biodegradable materials and supporting circular economy initiatives may provide sustainable alternatives to conventional plastics.

5.2.2 Public awareness and education

As awareness of MP pollution continues to grow, the role of effective public education and informed societal engagement becomes increasingly critical. Public awareness is not merely a matter of disseminating facts; it requires a well-orchestrated effort to translate complex scientific evidence into accessible knowledge, motivating informed decision-making and sustainable behavior changes across populations. Given this evolving understanding, effective communication strategies become paramount to fostering awareness and empowering individuals to participate proactively in mitigation efforts.

Educational initiatives should prioritize accurate, evidence-based information that addresses both the scientific uncertainties and confirmed risks. Clear communication must carefully avoid alarmism, which could lead to public disengagement or undue anxiety. Instead, it should underscore actionable steps individuals can take to reduce personal and environmental exposure. These steps include minimizing consumption of single-use plastics, supporting policies aimed at waste reduction, recycling initiatives, and encouraging public engagement in cleanup programs. Educational messaging should be grounded in verifiable science, transparently acknowledging current limitations and areas where further research is necessary, thereby building trust and encouraging continuous learning. Interactive and participatory approaches, such as student-led environmental audits, local community projects, and citizen science initiatives, can significantly enhance the effectiveness of these educational interventions by promoting hands-on engagement and fostering a personal connection to the issue. Professional development and continuous medical education programs must incorporate up-to-date findings on MPs, thereby enabling clinicians to guide patients toward informed health and lifestyle decisions.

To sum up, addressing the challenge of MPs and human health through public awareness and education necessitates a multifaceted, evidence-based approach. Clear communication, educational integration, digital media engagement, multidisciplinary collaboration, informed policy-making, and rigorous evaluation constitute essential components of a successful strategy. By empowering communities through knowledge, fostering proactive participation, and cultivating sustainable behaviors, society can significantly mitigate MP pollution's potential health impacts and contribute positively to both human health and environmental resilience.

5.3 Directions for future research

Future studies of MP-induced male reproductive toxicity should fill critical knowledge gaps by encompassing mechanistic, molecular, environmental, and translational studies [162]. At the mechanistic level, the definition of adverse outcome pathways through quantification of thresholds of oxidative stress (e.g., deformity of sperm mediated through ROS via p38 MAPK) and epigenetic mechanisms (e.g., histone modifications and DNA methylation in spermatogonia following low-dose, long-duration exposure to MP) can be used to explain the nexus of transgenerational infertility [162]. Comparative particle-sized (e.g., 20 nm *vs.* 1 μm MPs) exposure experiments and real-life co-exposures (e.g. PET, BPA and heavy metals) should provide a better picture of the exposure dynamics, to define the synergistic toxic effects [86].

5.3.1 Identification of sensitive biomarkers

Detection and, in particular, the development of biomarkers and real-time monitoring is critical to MP detection, such as mass spectrometry of MP metabolites in seminal plasma and Raman micro-spectroscopy of *in situ* tissue imaging.

Superparamagnetic iron oxide nanoparticles (e.g., Fe_3O_4, 60 nm) achieve 89% removal efficiency for MPs in complex biological fluids (e.g., semen) through magnetic sequestration. Their high surface-area-to-volume ratio and functionalizability enable targeted binding and external magnetic recovery of MPs [163]. The outcome of the work undertaken on MPs may be used in regulatory constructs by setting thresholds of toxicological concern through benchmark dose modeling and the identification of hotspots of MP emissions through lifecycle analysis [105]. New technologies such as human testis organ-on-chip technologies and multi-omics combination (e.g., epigenomics of sperm and gut, metagenomics and proteomics) will support species extrapolation precision and assist in the identification of genetically vulnerable populations (e.g., GSTM1 null genotype), leading to individualized risk evaluation and intervention [164].

5.3.2 Prospective cohort and multi-center studies

Experimental-to-human health risk translation requires the detailed, prospective cohort and multi-center studies precisely quantifying both: MP exposures and reproductive outcomes in a heterogeneous population. They need to use specific, high-sensitivity methods of analysis of MP biomarkers, well-characterized endpoints in male infertility, and adherence to extended follow-up to measure the late or latent effects [165]. Multi-center cooperation will increase the protection strength, universality, and geographical spread of research outcomes, which will aid solid risk appraisal, regulation principle, and prevention methodology [166]. No information on the candidate molecular biomarkers identified in animal and organoid models can be fully considered valid except with cohort studies that can validate its clinical attention and relevance [151].

The longitudinal cohort studies play an important role in investigating the chronological effect of chronic exposure of MPs on the living system [167]. Such studies would involve repeated measures of exposure to MP and health outcomes measured and adjusted to confounding variables in order to determine causality. Combining biomarkers denoting inflammation and bio-accumulation might deliver some insights on the mechanistic pathways. Interdisciplinary and collaboration between environmental science, toxicology, and epidemiology through collective work is required to provide key solutions to these future directions comprehensively [167].

6. Conclusions

6.1 Summary of current evidence

The pervasive presence of MPs in environmental and human systems necessitates urgent attention due to their potential threat to male reproductive health. The existing body of evidence underscores a disturbing trend, with MPs influencing reproductive function through multiple mechanisms, including oxidative stress, disruption of the BTB, and endocrine interference. These effects, compounded by the widespread nature of MP exposure via ingestion, inhalation, and dermal contact, pose significant risks to male fertility, with epidemiological studies revealing associations with impaired sperm quality and male infertility.

Animal studies have elucidated dose-response relationships and raised concerns about potential transgenerational effects, also underlining the importance of a profound knowledge of MP toxicity. Despite these findings, the field remains nascent, and critical knowledge gaps persist, particularly regarding long-term exposure outcomes and the cumulative effects of MPs on reproductive health.

6.2 Research and policy priorities

The mounting evidence of MP exposure as a significant threat to male reproductive health necessitates a strategic research agenda and policy framework to address this emerging public health concern. Future research must prioritize the following key areas to deepen our understanding of MPs' effects on reproductive function:

1. Mechanisms of toxicity: Further investigation is needed into the molecular mechanisms by which MPs induce oxidative stress, disrupt the BTB, and interfere with endocrine regulation. A more comprehensive understanding of these pathways is essential to identify potential biomarkers of exposure and susceptibility.

2. Dose-response and long-term effects: There is a need to better delineate the dose-response relationships between MP exposure and male reproductive outcomes. Longitudinal studies should be conducted to assess the cumulative effects of chronic exposure, including potential transgenerational impacts on reproductive health.

3. Epidemiological research: Expanded cohort studies are crucial to establish more robust epidemiological evidence linking MP exposure to adverse reproductive outcomes in human populations. This includes evaluating the impact on sperm quality, fertility rates, and overall male reproductive health across diverse demographic groups.

4. Risk assessment and regulation: Policymakers must work with researchers to establish clear guidelines for safe levels of MP exposure, particularly in food, water, and air. Regulatory frameworks should be developed to limit the environmental release of MPs, with a focus on reducing their prevalence in ecosystems and minimizing human exposure through public health initiatives. The interpretable machine learning (IML) models should be employed to predict chemical toxicities accurately, efficiently, and transparently, thereby enhancing chemical risk assessment and safety testing. While advanced ML and deep learning algorithms offer considerable predictive accuracy, their inherent "black-box" nature impedes interpretability, crucial for acceptance and application in toxicology.

   Given the established relevance of these computational techniques in evaluating toxicity mechanisms, this work provides foundational methodologies that are particularly applicable to investigating the detrimental effects of MP exposure on male reproductive health. By employing computational models informed by pathway-based toxicological mechanisms, researchers can better elucidate the intricate processes through which MPs may compromise male fertility, thus enhancing the precision and efficacy of health risk assessments and interventions.

5. Public health interventions: Since MPs may have a significant impact on male fertility, there must be campaigns which will create awareness on the danger of exposure to MPs and also help individuals prevent the exposure to these MPs. To mitigate these effects, there should be strategies, such as minimizing the amount of plastic waste, developing better waste disposal systems, and promoting the use of safer alternatives to plastic products.

6.3 Call for coordinated global action

Moving forward, it is imperative to prioritize targeted research to elucidate the precise molecular pathways through which MPs exert their effects on male reproductive function. Concurrently, public health initiatives must be launched to reduce exposure to these pollutants and mitigate their adverse impacts. A coordinated global response is crucial to establish regulatory frameworks that limit MPs' environmental presence and safeguard human health. Collaborative efforts across research institutions, policymakers, and environmental agencies are essential to address this emerging public health challenge effectively.

6.4 Specific mandatory regulative measures for calls for regulatory interventions

6.4.1 Wastewater treatment plant upgrades

The introduction of advanced filtration technologies in the work of wastewater treatment plants can help limit MP capture [168].

6.4.2 Uniform the plastic product design standards

Create international guidelines on the content of MP in consumer products [169]. Plastic product design with an aim of re-use and recycling of products and the development of research of biodegradable substitutes to plastics should be encouraged [153].

6.4.3 Risk assessment and safe exposure levels

Risk assessment studies should be conducted which will determine the threshold levels of MPs in the outer environments, such as water, air, and soil [155].

6.4.4 Extended producer responsibility (EPR) programs

Launch EPR programs to get involved and handle plastic waste effectively beginning at the manufacturing stage right through to final disposal [169].

6.4.5 International regulatory environment

Some of the countries and areas already started to introduce regulations about MPs [170]. Some countries prohibited the use of MPs in some special forms. Microbeads have been prohibited in rinse-off cosmetics in the United States and Canada. Some plastic products are also banned in China. World state forms develop or design new legislature and regulations to confront MPs, with the EU being at the head [170].

6.5 Mitigation strategies

6.5.1 Green infrastructure

Since MPs are found in urban storm water run offs, using green infrastructure to urban stormwater management is practical to minimize MP contamination in the water [168].

6.5.2 Source reduction

Mitigate the MP pollution by implementing measures such as reduction in waste and a better practice of waste management [171]. Decrease the use of plastic and enhance the waste disposal mechanisms [171]. Encourage the use of biodegradable materials [171].

6.5.3 Advanced oxidation processes

Decompose the pollutants such as tetracycline using the UV/peroxydisulfate processes with mariculture wastewater. UV/PS treatment performed 30 min later resulted in the 95.73% removal of tetracycline in 5 mg/L dosage [172].

6.5.4 Innovative materials

Find out how to take the plasticizers out of the secondary wastewater effluent using flexible nanocatalysts [173].

6.5.5 Bioremediation

Photosynthetic living organisms can be used to bioremediate MPs within both aquatic and terrestrial environments [174] or to mitigate MP contamination. The rate of microbial breakdown can be increased [175].

Acknowledgements

This work was financially supported by the National Natural Science Foundation of China (grant no. 81872584), the Natural Science Foundation of Shenzhen (JCYJ20210324093211030), Key R&D and Promotion Projects (Scientific and Technological Research) of Henan Province (grant no. 252102310075), Sanming Project of Medicine in Shenzhen (SZSM202211009), and Interdisciplinary Research for First-class Discipline Construction Project of Henan University (2019YLXKJC04).

Conflict of interest

The authors declare no conflict of interest.

Author details

Zubair Muhammad[1,2], Qiming Yang[1,3] and Nan Liu[1,2,3]*

1 Institute of Environment and Health, South China Hospital, Medical School, Shenzhen University, Shenzhen, P. R. China

2 Basic Medical Sciences, School of Biomedical Engineering (Medicine), Shenzhen University, Shenzhen, P. R. China

3 Department of Environmental Toxicology, School of Public Health, Shandong Second Medical University, Weifang, P. R. China

*Address all correspondence to: nanliu@szu.edu.cn

References

[1] Mo J et al. Developmental origins of adult diseases. Medical Review. 2022;**2**(5):450-470

[2] Feng Y et al. A systematic review of the impacts of exposure to micro- and nano-plastics on human tissue accumulation and health. Eco-Environment & Health. 2023;**2**(4):195-207

[3] Qian N et al. Rapid single-particle chemical imaging of nanoplastics by SRS microscopy. Proceedings of the National Academy of Sciences. 2024;**121**(3):e2300582121

[4] Kaandorp MLA et al. Global mass of buoyant marine plastics dominated by large long-lived debris. Nature Geoscience. 2023;**16**(8):689-694

[5] Hirt N, Body-Malapel M. Immunotoxicity and intestinal effects of nano- and microplastics: A review of the literature. Particle and Fibre Toxicology. 2020;**17**(1):57

[6] Zhao X et al. Airborne microplastics: Occurrence, sources, fate, risks and mitigation. Science of the Total Environment. 2023;**858**:159943

[7] Marfella R et al. Microplastics and nanoplastics in atheromas and cardiovascular events. New England Journal of Medicine. 2024;**390**(10):900-910

[8] Domenech J et al. Interactions of polystyrene nanoplastics with in vitro models of the human intestinal barrier. Archives of Toxicology. 2020;**94**(9):2997-3012

[9] Huang W, Xia X. Element cycling with micro(nano)plastics. Science. 2024;**385**(6712):933-935

[10] Vdovchenko A, Resmini M. Mapping microplastics in humans: Analysis of polymer types, and shapes in food and drinking water—A systematic review. International Journal of Molecular Sciences. 2024;**25**(13):7074

[11] Dawson AL, Li JY, Kroon FJ. Plastics for dinner: Store-bought seafood, but not wild-caught from the great barrier reef, as a source of microplastics to human consumers. Environmental Advances. 2022;**8**:100249

[12] Yang Z et al. Human microplastics exposure and potential health risks to target organs by different routes: A review. Current Pollution Reports. 2023;**9**(3):468-485

[13] Kannan K, Vimalkumar K. A review of human exposure to microplastics and insights into microplastics as obesogens. Frontiers in Endocrinology. 2021;**12**:724989

[14] Ageel HK, Harrad S, Abdallah MA-E. Occurrence, human exposure, and risk of microplastics in the indoor environment. Environmental Science: Processes & Impacts. 2022;**24**(1):17-31

[15] Sun A, Wang W-X. Human exposure to microplastics and its associated health risks. Environment & Health. 2023;**1**(3):139-149

[16] Yee MS-L et al. Impact of microplastics and nanoplastics on human health. Nanomaterials. 2021;**11**(2):496

[17] Prathipa R et al. Impact of microplastics on human health: A comprehensive review. Journal of Preventive, Diagnostic and Treatment Strategies in Medicine. 2024;**3**(2):76-84

[18] Tang KHD et al. Health risk of human exposure to microplastics: A review. Environmental Chemistry Letters. 2024;**22**(3):1155-1183

[19] Zhu L et al. Tissue accumulation of microplastics and potential health risks in human. Science of the Total Environment. 2024;**915**:170004

[20] Wang M et al. The hidden threat: Unraveling the impact of microplastics on reproductive health. Science of the Total Environment. 2024;**935**:173177

[21] Kumar N, Mangla M. Microplastics and impaired male reproductive health-exploring biological pathways of harm: A narrative review. Biology of Reproduction. 2025;**112**(6):1028-1038

[22] Ali W et al. A critical review on male-female reproductive and developmental toxicity induced by micro-plastics and nano-plastics through different signaling pathways. Chemico-Biological Interactions. 2024;**394**:110976

[23] Hunt CF, Lin WH, Voulvoulis N. Evaluating alternatives to plastic microbeads in cosmetics. Nature Sustainability. 2020;**4**(4):366-372

[24] Yong CQY, Valiyaveettil S, Tang BL. Toxicity of microplastics and nanoplastics in mammalian systems. International Journal of Environmental Research and Public Health. 2020;**17**(5):1509

[25] Napper IE, Thompson RC. Release of synthetic microplastic plastic fibres from domestic washing machines: Effects of fabric type and washing conditions. Marine Pollution Bulletin. 2016;**112**(1-2):39-45

[26] Hossain MI et al. Fibrous microplastics release from textile production phases: A brief review of current challenges and applied research directions. Materials (Basel). 2025;**18**(11):2513

[27] Kounina A et al. The global apparel industry is a significant yet overlooked source of plastic leakage. Nature Communications. 2024;**15**(1):5022

[28] Law KL et al. Untangling the chemical complexity of plastics to improve life cycle outcomes. Nature Reviews Materials. 2024;**9**(9):657-667

[29] Sieber G et al. Microbial community shifts induced by plastic and zinc as substitutes of tire abrasion. Scientific Reports. 2022;**12**(1):18684

[30] Juntarasakul O et al. Weave structures of polyester fabric affect the tensile strength and microplastic fiber emission during the laundry process. Scientific Reports. 2025;**15**(1):2272

[31] Lavers JL et al. Significant plastic accumulation on the Cocos (Keeling) Islands, Australia. Scientific Reports. 2019;**9**(1):7102

[32] Ragusa A et al. Raman microspectroscopy detection and characterisation of microplastics in human breastmilk. Polymers (Basel). 2022;**14**(13):2700

[33] Barceló D, Picó Y, Alfarhan AH. Microplastics: Detection in human samples, cell line studies, and health impacts. Environmental Toxicology and Pharmacology. 2023;**101**:104204

[34] Gautam R et al. Evaluation of potential toxicity of polyethylene microplastics on human derived cell lines. Science of the Total Environment. 2022;**838**(Pt 2):156089

[35] Aschner M. Mind over microplastics—What we still don't

know. Nature Reviews. Neurology. 2025;**4**(6):1900022

[36] Codrington J et al. Detection of microplastics in the human penis. International Journal of Impotence Research. 2025;**37**(5):377-383

[37] Prata JC et al. Environmental exposure to microplastics: An overview on possible human health effects. Science of the Total Environment. 2020;**702**:134455

[38] Revel M, Châtel A, Mouneyrac C. Micro(nano)plastics: A threat to human health? Current Opinion in Environmental Science & Health. 2018;**1**:17-23

[39] Campanale C et al. A detailed review study on potential effects of microplastics and additives of concern on human health. International Journal of Environmental Research and Public Health. 2020;**17**(4):1212

[40] Wright SL, Kelly FJ. Plastic and human health: A micro issue? Environmental Science & Technology. 2017;**51**(12):6634-6647

[41] Nihart AJ et al. Bioaccumulation of microplastics in decedent human brains. Nature Medicine. 2025;**31**(4):1114-1119

[42] Microplastics in drinking-water. ISBN978-92-4-151619-8

[43] Thapliyal C et al. Mechanistic insight into potential toxic effects of microplastics and nanoplastics on human health. Discover Applied Sciences. 2025;7(6):645

[44] Xia X et al. Reproductive toxicity and cross-generational effect of polyethylene microplastics in Paramisgurnus dabryanus. Chemosphere. 2023;**313**:137440

[45] Ijaz MU et al. Mitigative potential of kaempferide against polyethylene microplastics induced testicular damage by activating Nrf-2/Keap-1 pathway. Ecotoxicology and Environmental Safety. 2024;**269**:115746

[46] Jin H et al. Chronic exposure to polystyrene microplastics induced male reproductive toxicity and decreased testosterone levels via the LH-mediated LHR/cAMP/PKA/StAR pathway. Particle and Fibre Toxicology. 2022;**19**(1):13

[47] Wu D et al. Long-term exposure to polystyrene microplastics triggers premature testicular aging. Particle and Fibre Toxicology. 2023;**20**(1):35

[48] Takalani NB et al. Role of oxidative stress in male infertility. Reproduction and Fertility. 2023;**4**(3):e230024

[49] Shipp A et al. Acrylamide: Review of toxicity data and dose-response analyses for cancer and noncancer effects. Critical Reviews in Toxicology. 2006;**36**(6-7):481-608

[50] Wei Y et al. Polystyrene microplastics disrupt the blood-testis barrier integrity through ROS-mediated imbalance of mTORC1 and mTORC2. Environmental Pollution. 2021;**289**:117904

[51] Zubair M, Ahmad M, Qureshi Z. Review on arsenic-induced toxicity in male reproductive system and its amelioration. Andrologia. 2017;**49**(9):e12791

[52] Zhou D et al. Di-n-butyl phthalate (DBP) exposure induces oxidative damage in testes of adult rats. Systems Biology in Reproductive Medicine. 2010;**56**(6):413-419

[53] Alahmar AT. Role of oxidative stress in male infertility: An updated review.

Journal of Human Reproductive Sciences. 2019;**12**(1):4-18

[54] Khosrowbeygi A, Zarghami N. Fatty acid composition of human spermatozoa and seminal plasma levels of oxidative stress biomarkers in subfertile males. Prostaglandins, Leukotrienes and Essential Fatty Acids. 2007;**77**(2):117-121

[55] Płuciennik K et al. Important factors affecting induction of cell death, oxidative stress and DNA damage by nano-and microplastic particles in vitro. Cells. 2024;**13**(9):768

[56] Lord T, Aitken RJ. Fertilization stimulates 8-hydroxy-2′-deoxyguanosine repair and antioxidant activity to prevent mutagenesis in the embryo. Developmental Biology. 2015;**406**(1):1-13

[57] Jiang B, Yang D, Peng H. Environmental toxins and reproductive health: Unraveling the effects on sertoli cells and the blood–testis barrier in animals. Biology of Reproduction. 2024;**111**(5):977-986

[58] Li S et al. Polystyrene microplastics induce blood–testis barrier disruption regulated by the MAPK-Nrf2 signaling pathway in rats. Environmental Science and Pollution Research. 2021;**28**(35):47921-47931

[59] Zheng S, Jiang L, Qiu L. The effects of fine particulate matter on the blood-testis barrier and its potential mechanisms. Reviews on Environmental Health. 2024;**39**(2):233-249

[60] Wong CH, Cheng CY. The blood-testis barrier: Its biology, regulation, and physiological role in spermatogenesis. Current Topics in Developmental Biology. 2005;**71**:263-296

[61] Zhang Y et al. Phthalates (PAEs) and reproductive toxicity: Hypothalamic-pituitary-gonadal (HPG) axis aspects. Journal of Hazardous Materials. 2023;**459**:132182

[62] Jin H et al. Reproductive toxicity of chronic exposure to polystyrene microplastics and the molecular mechanism of decrease in testosterone levels in male mice. Preprint from Research Square. Jul 2021. PPR: PPR371613

[63] Urli S et al. Impact of microplastics and nanoplastics on livestock health: An emerging risk for reproductive efficiency. Animals. 2023;**13**(7):1132

[64] Li L et al. Hormone regulation in testicular development and function. International Journal of Molecular Sciences. 2024;**25**(11):5805

[65] Lin P-H et al. Downregulation of testosterone production through luteinizing hormone receptor regulation in male rats exposed to 17α-ethynylestradiol. Scientific Reports. 2020;**10**(1):1576

[66] Yang L et al. DEHP-mediated oxidative stress leads to impaired testosterone synthesis in Leydig cells through the cAMP/PKA/SF-1/StAR pathway. Environmental Pollution. 2025;**366**:125503

[67] Qu J et al. Polystyrene microplastics trigger testosterone decline via GPX1. Science of the Total Environment. 2024;**947**:174536

[68] Liu Y, Li X, Xiong Y. Chronic polystyrene microplastic exposure reduces testosterone levels in mice through mitochondrial oxidative stress and BAX/BCL2-mediated apoptosis. Toxics. 2024;**12**(8):561

[69] Grillo G et al. Polystyrene microplastics impair the functions

of cultured mouse Leydig (TM3) and Sertoli (TM4) cells by inducing mitochondrial-endoplasmic reticulum damage. Ecotoxicology and Environmental Safety. 2024;**274**:116202

[70] Zhao Q et al. Polystyrene microplastics impaired the function of leydig cells via GRP78/PERK/CHOP mediated endoplasmic reticulum stress in vivo and in vitro. Ecotoxicology and Environmental Safety. 2025;**292**:117985

[71] Kim SanWoong KS et al. Cistanches herba induces testis cytotoxicity in male mice. Bulletin of Environmental Contamination and Toxicology. Jan 2012;**88**(1):112-117

[72] O'Shaughnessy PJ. Hormonal control of germ cell development and spermatogenesis. In: Seminars in Cell & Developmental Biology. Elsevier; 29 May 2014:55-65

[73] Sofikitis N et al. Hormonal regulation of spermatogenesis and spermiogenesis. The Journal of Steroid Biochemistry and Molecular Biology. 2008;**109**(3-5):323-330

[74] Ye J et al. Understanding the impact of nanoplastics on reproductive health: Exposure pathways, mechanisms, and implications. Toxicology. 2024;**504**:153792

[75] Kauts S et al. The evidence of in-vivo and in-vitro studies on microplastic and nano plastic toxicity in mammals: A possible threat for an upcoming generation? Physics and Chemistry of the Earth, Parts A/B/C. 2023;**132**:103511

[76] Zhang Z et al. Reproductive toxicity of cadmium stress in male animals. Toxicology. 2024;**504**:153787

[77] Zhang X et al. Damaged spermatogenic cells induce inflammatory gene expression in mouse Sertoli cells through the activation of toll-like receptors 2 and 4. Molecular and Cellular Endocrinology. 2013;**365**(2):162-173

[78] Kumar N et al. Microplastics–a growing concern as carcinogens in cancer etiology: Emphasis on biochemical and molecular mechanisms. Cell Biochemistry and Biophysics. 2024;**82**(4):3109-3121

[79] Hou L et al. Polystyrene microplastics induce apoptosis in chicken testis via crosstalk between NF-κB and Nrf2 pathways. Comparative Biochemistry and Physiology Part C: Toxicology & Pharmacology. 2022;**262**:109444

[80] Chen S et al. Targeting TBK1 attenuates ocular inflammation in uveitis by antagonizing NF-κB signaling. Clinical Immunology. 2023;**246**:109210

[81] Li N, Wang T, Han D. Structural, cellular and molecular aspects of immune privilege in the testis. Frontiers in Immunology. 2012;**3**:152

[82] Zhang Q et al. Microplastics induced inflammation in the spleen of developmental Japanese quail (Coturnix japonica) via ROS-mediated p38 MAPK and TNF signaling pathway activation1. Environmental Pollution. 2024;**341**:122891

[83] Yao K et al. Inflammation—The role of TRPA1 channel. Frontiers in Physiology. 2023;**14**:1093925

[84] Ijaz MU et al. Dose-dependent effect of polystyrene microplastics on the testicular tissues of the male Sprague Dawley rats. Dose-Response. 2021;**19**(2):15593258211019882

[85] Deng Y et al. Polystyrene microplastics affect the reproductive performance of male mice and

lipid homeostasis in their offspring. Environmental Science & Technology Letters. 2022;**9**(9):752-757

[86] Fang Q, Wang C, Xiong Y. Polystyrene microplastics induce male reproductive toxicity in mice by activating spermatogonium mitochondrial oxidative stress and apoptosis. Chemico-Biological Interactions. 2024;**396**:111043

[87] Jin H et al. Polystyrene microplastics induced male reproductive toxicity in mice. Journal of Hazardous Materials. 2021;**401**:123430

[88] Islam MS, Islam MM. Polystyrene microplastic exposure in mice: Oxidative stress-induced testicular damage, AR gene suppression, and histopathological alterations. Journal of Experimental and Laboratory Medicine. 2024;**11**(3):e70393

[89] Gao L et al. The male reproductive toxicity after nanoplastics and microplastics exposure: Sperm quality and changes of different cells in testis. Ecotoxicology and Environmental Safety. 2023;**267**:115618

[90] Dou Y et al. Lactating exposure to microplastics at the dose of infants ingested during artificial feeding induced reproductive toxicity in female mice and their offspring. Science of the Total Environment. 2024;**949**:174972

[91] Chen H et al. Transgenerational reproductive toxicity induced by carboxyl and amino charged microplastics at environmental concentrations in Caenorhabditis elegans: Involvement of histone methylation. Science of the Total Environment. 2024;**949**:175132

[92] Wen S et al. Microplastics-perturbed gut microbiota triggered the testicular disorder in male mice: Via fecal microbiota transplantation. Environmental Pollution. 2022;**309**:119789

[93] Skinner MK et al. Alterations in sperm DNA methylation, non-coding RNA and histone retention associate with DDT-induced epigenetic transgenerational inheritance of disease. Epigenetics & Chromatin. 2018;**11**:1-24

[94] Ben Maamar M et al. Alterations in sperm DNA methylation, non-coding RNA expression, and histone retention mediate vinclozolin-induced epigenetic transgenerational inheritance of disease. Environmental. Epigenetics. 2018;**4**(2):dvy010

[95] Li C et al. Effects of particulate matter on the risk of gestational hypertensive disorders and their progression. Environmental Science & Technology. 2023;**57**(12):4930-4939

[96] Su Y-F et al. Associations between short-term and long-term exposure to particulate matter and preterm birth. Chemosphere. 2023;**313**:137431

[97] Chris R. Plastic pollution and potential solutions. Sci Progress-Uk. 2018;**101**(**3**):207-260

[98] Ragusa A et al. Plasticenta: First evidence of microplastics in human placenta. Environment International. 2021;**146**:106274

[99] Zhao Q et al. Detection and characterization of microplastics in the human testis and semen. Science of the Total Environment. 2023;**877**:162713

[100] Zhang C et al. Association of mixed exposure to microplastics with sperm dysfunction: A multi-site study in China. eBioMedicine. 2024;**108**:105369

[101] Wen Y et al. The potential mechanisms involved in the disruption of

spermatogenesis in mice by nanoplastics and microplastics. Biomedicine. 2024;**12**(8):1714

[102] Zhang Y et al. Association between ambient PM1 and semen quality: A cross-sectional study of 27,854 men in China. Environment International. 2023;**175**:107919

[103] Lin Z et al. Microplastics from face mask impairs sperm motility. Marine Pollution Bulletin. 2024;**203**:116422

[104] Mottola F et al. Reproductive cytotoxic and genotoxic impact of polystyrene microplastic on paracentrotus lividus spermatozoa. Current Research in Toxicology. 2024;**6**:100173

[105] Chen Y et al. Occurrence, toxicity and removal of polystyrene microplastics and nanoplastics in human sperm. Environmental Chemistry Letters. 2024;**22**(5):2159-2165

[106] Henkel R, Selvaraju V, Baskaran S. Environmental contaminants and male infertility: Effects and mechanisms. Andrologia. 2021;**53**(1):e13646

[107] Belladelli F, Muncey W, Eisenberg ML. Reproduction as a window for health in men. Fertility and Sterility. 2023;**120**(3):429-437

[108] Carrageta DF et al. Signatures of metabolic diseases on spermatogenesis and testicular metabolism. Nature Reviews Urology. 2024;**21**(8):477-494

[109] Panga MJ, Zhao Y. Male reproductive toxicity of antifouling chemicals: Insights into oxidative stress-induced infertility and molecular mechanisms of zinc pyrithione (ZPT). Antioxidants. 2024;**13**(2):173

[110] Johannessen C, Helm P, Metcalfe CD. Detection of selected tire wear compounds in urban receiving waters. Environmental Pollution. 2021;**287**:117659

[111] Biggs SN et al. Lifestyle and environmental risk factors for unexplained male infertility: Study protocol for Australian male infertility exposure (AMIE), a case–control study. Reproductive Health. 2023;**20**(1):32

[112] Pandruvada S et al. Lack of trusted diagnostic tools for undetermined male infertility. Journal of Assisted Reproduction and Genetics. 2021;**38**:265-276

[113] Zhao M et al. Disturbance of mitochondrial dynamics led to spermatogenesis disorder in mice exposed to polystyrene micro-and nanoplastics. Environmental Pollution. 2024;**362**:124935

[114] Zhou Y et al. Gut microbiota combined with metabolome dissects long-term nanoplastics exposure-induced disturbed spermatogenesis. Ecotoxicology and Environmental Safety. 2023;**267**:115626

[115] Gao Q et al. Tracking of realistic nanoplastics in complicated matrices by iridium element labeling and inductively coupled plasma mass spectroscopy. Journal of Hazardous Materials. 2022;**424**:127628

[116] Kwak JI, An Y-J. Microplastic digestion generates fragmented nanoplastics in soils and damages earthworm spermatogenesis and coelomocyte viability. Journal of Hazardous Materials. 2021;**402**:124034

[117] Sun Z et al. Exposure to nanoplastics induces mitochondrial impairment and cytomembrane destruction in Leydig cells. Ecotoxicology and Environmental Safety. 2023;**255**:114796

[118] He Y, Yin R. The reproductive and transgenerational toxicity of microplastics and nanoplastics: A threat to mammalian fertility in both sexes. Journal of Applied Toxicology. 2024;**44**(1):66-85

[119] Yu Y et al. Carboxyl-modified polystyrene microplastics induces neurotoxicity by affecting dopamine, glutamate, serotonin, and GABA neurotransmission in *Caenorhabditis elegans*. Journal of Hazardous Materials. 2023;**445**:130543

[120] Slob W et al. The use of canonical dose–response models for benchmark dose analysis of continuous toxicological data. Critical Reviews in Toxicology. 2025;**55**(4):437-461

[121] Keshtkar E, Kudsk P, Mesgaran MB. Perspective: Common errors in dose–response analysis and how to avoid them. Pest Management Science. 2021;**77**(6):2599-2608

[122] Yuan W et al. The male reproductive toxicity after 5-fluorouracil exposure: DNA damage, oxidative stress, and mitochondrial dysfunction in vitro and in vivo. Ecotoxicology and Environmental Safety. 2024;**278**:116465

[123] Jin H et al. Chronic exposure to polystyrene microplastics induced LHR reduction and decreased testosterone levels through NF-κB pathway. Environmental Pollution. 2024;**358**:124543

[124] Jiang J et al. Animal models: An essential tool to dissect the heterogeneity of chronic obstructive pulmonary disease. Journal of Translational Internal Medicine. 2023;**11**(1):4-10

[125] Cui Y, Chen Y. Blood eosinophils in chronic obstructive pulmonary disease: A potential biomarker. Journal of Translational Internal Medicine. 2023;**11**(3):193-197

[126] Zhang J et al. Prospective prenatal cell-free DNA screening for genetic conditions of heterogenous etiologies. Nature Medicine. 2024;**30**(2):470-479

[127] Tripathy B, Dash A, Das AP. Detection of environmental microfiber pollutants through vibrational spectroscopic techniques: Recent advances of environmental monitoring and future prospects. Critical Reviews in Analytical Chemistry. 2024;**54**(7):1925-1935

[128] Resurreccion EP, Fong K-W. The integration of metabolomics with other omics: Insights into understanding prostate cancer. Metabolites. 2022;**12**(6):488

[129] Sakib S et al. Generation of porcine testicular organoids with testis specific architecture using microwell culture. Journal of Visualized Experiments (JoVE). 2019;**152**:e60387

[130] Yang Y et al. In vitro reconstitution of the hormone-responsive testicular organoids from murine primary testicular cells. Biofabrication. 2022;**15**(1):015001

[131] Enyoh CE et al. The plastic within: Microplastics invading human organs and bodily fluids systems. Environments. 2023;**10**(11):194

[132] Malafaia G, Marinho T, da Luz A, da Costa P, Araújo MA, Ahmed I, et al. Novel methodology for identification and quantification of microplastics in biological samples. Environmental Pollution. 2022;**292**:118466

[133] Fiore D, Cristina FC, Russo MV, Avino P. Are microplastics a macro issue? A review on the sources of

contamination, analytical challenges and impact on human health of microplastics in food. Foods. 2023;**12**:3915

[134] Han X-L, Jiang N-J, Hata T, Choi J, Yan-Jun D, Wang Y-J. Deep learning based approach for automated characterization of large marine microplastic particles. Marine Environmental Research. 2023;**183**:105829

[135] Baert Y et al. Primary human testicular cells self-organize into organoids with testicular properties. Stem Cell Reports. 2017;**8**(1):30-38

[136] Saha U et al. Detrimental consequences of micropolymers associated plasticizers on endocrinal disruption. Materials Today Bio. 2024;**27**:101139

[137] Rivera-Rivera DM, Quintanilla-Villanueva GE, Luna-Moreno D, Sánchez-Álvarez A, Rodríguez-Delgado JM, Cedillo-González EI, et al. Exploring innovative approaches for the analysis of micro-and nanoplastics: Breakthroughs in (bio) sensing techniques. Biosensors. 2025;**15**:44

[138] Dey T. Microplastic pollutant detection by surface enhanced Raman spectroscopy (SERS): A mini-review. Nanotechnology for Environmental Engineering. 2023;**8**:41-48

[139] Shen X et al. Multi-omics microsampling for the profiling of lifestyle-associated changes in health. Nature Biomedical Engineering. 2024;**8**(1):11-29

[140] Wang H et al. *Ginkgo biloba* extract alleviates deltamethrin-induced testicular injury by upregulating SKP2 and inhibiting Beclin1-independent autophagy. Phytomedicine. 2024;**135**:156245

[141] Zhang Y, Haiwen W, Li X, Liu H, An L. Promising indicators for monitoring microplastic pollution. Marine Pollution Bulletin. 2022;**182**:113952

[142] Xing R, Sun H, Xian D, Lin H, Qin S, Chen Z, et al. Enhanced degradation of microplastics during sludge composting via microbially-driven Fenton reaction. Journal of Hazardous Materials. 2023;**449**:131031

[143] Michalke B. Review about powerful combinations of advanced and hyphenated sample introduction techniques with inductively coupled plasma-mass spectrometry (ICP-MS) for elucidating trace element species in pathologic conditions on a molecular level. International Journal of Molecular Sciences. 2022;**23**(11):6109

[144] Zarfl C. Promising techniques and open challenges for microplastic identification and quantification in environmental matrices. Analytical and Bioanalytical Chemistry. 2019;**411**:3743-3756

[145] Esteves SC. Evolution of the World Health Organization semen analysis manual: Where are we? Nature Reviews Urology. 2022;**19**(7):439-446

[146] Yue Y et al. Multi-omics and gut microbiome: Unveiling the pathogenic mechanisms of early-life pesticide exposure. Pesticide Biochemistry and Physiology. 2024;**199**:105770

[147] Hu M et al. The effects of micro/Nano-plastics exposure on plants and their toxic mechanisms: A review from multi-omics perspectives. Journal of Hazardous Materials. 2024;**465**:133279

[148] Omolaoye TS et al. Omics and male infertility: Highlighting the

application of transcriptomic data. Life. 2022;**12**(2):280

[149] Podgrajsek R et al. Insight into the complexity of male infertility: A multi-omics review. Systems Biology in Reproductive Medicine. 2024;**70**(1):73-90

[150] Llavanera M et al. A systematic review identifying fertility biomarkers in semen: A clinical approach through omics to diagnose male infertility. Fertility and Sterility. 2022;**118**(2):291-313

[151] Vineis P, Chadeau-Hyam M. Integrating biomarkers into molecular epidemiological studies. Current Opinion in Oncology. 2011;**23**(1):100-105

[152] Sakib S, de Lima N, e Martins Lara, Brandon Christopher Huynh, and Ina Dobrinski. Organotypic rat testicular organoids for the study of testicular maturation and toxicology. Frontiers in Endocrinology. 2022;**13**:892342

[153] Samuel H, Makong F-D, Ori M. Green chemistry strategies for mitigating microplastic pollution in aquatic environments. Asian Journal of Environmental Research. 2024;**1**(2):73-82

[154] Kwak E, Peng G. Human-organoid-based in vitro modeling for environmental toxicology. Environmental Science & Technology Letters. 2024;**11**:503-510

[155] Mesnage R, Benbrook C. Use of the concept 'environmentally relevant level' in linking the results of pesticide toxicity studies to public health outcomes. All Life. 2023;**16**(1):2167872

[156] Huang Y, Dai Y, Li M, Guo L, Cao C, Huang Y, et al. Exposure to cadmium induces neuroinflammation and impairs ciliogenesis in hESC-derived 3D cerebral organoids. Science of the Total Environment. 2021;**797**:149043

[157] Li Y et al. A testicular microfluidic organ-on-a-chip for mimicking spermatogenic epithelium. Biomedical Materials. 2025;**20**(4):045009

[158] Nawab A et al. Human exposure to microplastics: A review on exposure routes and public health impacts. Journal of Hazardous Materials Advances. 2024;**16**:100487

[159] Dey S et al. Analytical approaches for quantifying and characterizing microplastics: Environmental impacts and bioaccumulation in aquatic systems. Green Analytical Chemistry. 2025;**12**:100191

[160] Li Y et al. Potential health impact of microplastics: A review of environmental distribution, human exposure, and toxic effects. Environ Health (Wash). 2023;**1**(4):249-257

[161] Abbasi S, Turner A. Human exposure to microplastics: A study in Iran. Journal of Hazardous Materials. 2021;**403**:123799

[162] Wang N et al. Recent advances in microplastics research: Impacts on mammalian sperm and reproductive health. Frontiers of Environmental Science & Engineering. 2025;**19**(6):79

[163] Zhang Y et al. Probiotics improve polystyrene microplastics-induced male reproductive toxicity in mice by alleviating inflammatory response. Ecotoxicology and Environmental Safety. 2023;**263**:115248

[164] Zhang X et al. Toxicity to the male reproductive system after exposure to polystyrene nanoplastics: A macrogenomic and metabolomic analysis. Toxics. 2024;**12**(8):531

[165] Hunt K et al. Exposure to microplastics and human reproductive outcomes: A systematic review. BJOG: An International Journal of Obstetrics & Gynaecology. 2024;**131**(5):675-683

[166] Chen G et al. An overview of analytical methods for detecting microplastics in the atmosphere. TrAC Trends in Analytical Chemistry. 2020;**130**:115981

[167] Ramesh K, Chellam PV, Sundaram B. Transport of layered and spherical microplastics in aqueous ecosystems: A review. Environmental Chemistry Letters. 2024;**22**(3):1221-1255

[168] Ahmad T et al. Microplastic mitigation in urban stormwater using green infrastructure: A review. Environmental Chemistry Letters. 2025;**23**:1-26

[169] Nafea TH et al. Status of management and mitigation of microplastic pollution. Critical Reviews in Environmental Science and Technology. 2024;**54**(24):1734-1756

[170] Halfar J et al. Disparities in methods used to determine microplastics in the aquatic environment: A review of legislation, sampling process and instrumental analysis. International Journal of Environmental Research and Public Health. 2021;**18**(14):7608

[171] Kumar A, Krishan G. Microplastic pollutants in aquatic ecosystems: Present and future challenges. MDPI. 2023:102

[172] Zhang Y et al. Insight in degradation of tetracycline in mariculture wastewater by ultraviolet/persulfate advanced oxidation process. Environmental Research. 2022;**212**:113324

[173] Yang W et al. Surface-catalyzed electro-Fenton with flexible nanocatalyst for removal of plasticizers from secondary wastewater effluent. Journal of Hazardous Materials. 2022;**435**:129023

[174] Barone GD et al. Harnessing photosynthetic microorganisms for enhanced bioremediation of microplastics: A comprehensive review. Environmental Science and Ecotechnology. 2024:100407

[175] Jain R et al. Microplastic pollution: Understanding microbial degradation and strategies for pollutant reduction. Science of the Total Environment. 2023;**905**:167098

Chapter 2

Role of Antioxidants in Male Semen Preservation

Daniel Ionut Berean

Abstract

A range of internal and external stressors increasingly challenges male fertility, among which oxidative stress, primarily driven by reactive oxygen species (ROS), plays a central role. The chapter explores the multifaceted impact of oxidative stress on male reproductive function, emphasizing its contribution to sperm damage, DNA fragmentation, and decreased fertility potential. Antioxidants, both conventional and emerging, have been shown to counteract these effects, offering therapeutic and preventive value. The discussion extends beyond standard treatments, integrating innovative advances such as nanotechnology-based delivery systems and mitochondria-targeted antioxidants. Personalized approaches, including biomarker-guided supplementation and genetic profiling, are proposed to optimize outcomes. Broader sociocultural and demographic disparities in access to antioxidant interventions are also addressed, highlighting the need for equitable healthcare strategies. Furthermore, the document connects antioxidant use to contemporary challenges such as delayed fatherhood, aging, and fertility preservation, with implications for clinical practice and public health policy. Novel applications, including antioxidants in cancer-related fertility care and cryopreservation, are considered.

Keywords: male fertility, oxidative stress, antioxidants, sperm quality, aging, delayed fatherhood, fertility preservation, nanotechnology

1. Introduction

Both intrinsic and extrinsic stressors can significantly influence male fertility, with ROS representing a major internal factor. Reactive oxygen species (ROS) are generated as natural by-products of aerobic metabolism, predominantly through the mitochondrial electron transport chain (ETC) [1, 2]. During this process, electrons are transferred sequentially across a series of protein complexes, a mechanism that can inadvertently result in ROS formation. Under certain metabolic conditions, such as shifts in substrate availability or disturbances in energy homeostasis, this electron transfer can become inefficient or backed up, disrupting the balance between electron donors and acceptors. Consequently, ROS production may increase as electrons prematurely react with alternative molecular targets instead of molecular oxygen. Due to their high chemical reactivity, ROS can oxidize a wide array of biomolecules, potentially altering their structure and impairing function [3].

Among the most commonly, produced ROS are superoxide anion (O_2), hydrogen peroxide (H_2O_2), and hydroxyl radicals (OH). Mitochondria, which are central to cellular energy production and signaling, generate both adenosine triphosphate (ATP) and ROS such as O_2 and H_2O_2 through electron transfer reactions. While ATP synthesis occurs *via* oxidative phosphorylation, superoxide arises from the one-electron reduction of molecular oxygen. This radical is rapidly dismutated to hydrogen peroxide by superoxide dismutase (SOD). Once considered merely detrimental by-products of respiration, superoxide and hydrogen peroxide are now recognized for their regulatory roles in diverse cellular pathways [2, 4].

Oxidative stress, arising from an imbalance between ROS production and antioxidant defense mechanisms, has been strongly associated with impaired sperm function and reduced fertility. Antioxidants mitigate oxidative damage by neutralizing free radicals, thereby preserving sperm integrity. The interplay between oxidative stress, ROS, and male reproductive health is complex; while excessive ROS levels can damage sperm DNA, membranes, and proteins, physiological levels are essential for normal sperm functions such as capacitation and the acrosome reaction. Moreover, ROS serve as secondary messengers in signaling pathways and modulate the activity of transcription factors involved in cellular development and differentiation. The basal ROS production, which accounts for approximately 2% of total mitochondrial activity even under optimal conditions, underscores their essential role in cellular physiology (**Figure 1**) [3, 5].

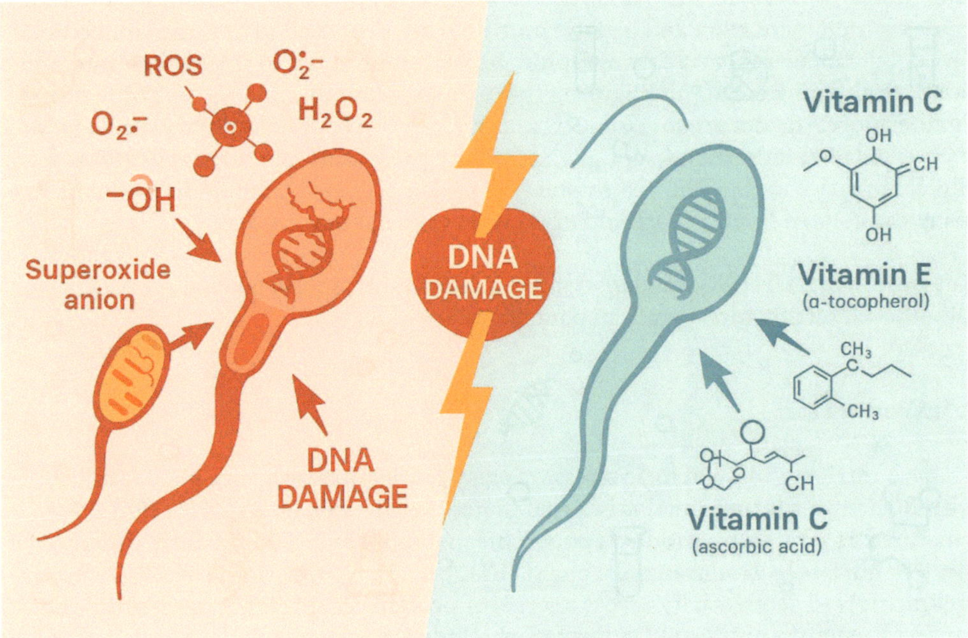

Figure 1.
Oxidative stress and antioxidant mechanisms in male fertility (on the left, excessive ROS generated by mitochondrial activity induce DNA fragmentation and impair sperm integrity. On the right, antioxidant molecules such as glutathione, vitamin C, and vitamin E neutralize ROS, preserving DNA stability and supporting sperm viability. The illustration highlights the critical balance between oxidative stress and antioxidant defenses in maintaining male reproductive potential).

2. Environmental and lifestyle factors that contribute to oxidative stress

2.1 Environmental factors

Environmental factors play a significant role in contributing to oxidative stress, particularly affecting male fertility and overall cellular health. Exposure to polluted environments, such as those containing airborne toxins, heavy metals, and industrial chemicals, has been shown to increase the burden of ROS [6]. Pollutants such as nitrogen dioxide, ozone, and fine particulate matter can penetrate deep into tissues, initiating oxidative reactions and compromising cellular structures. Similarly, heavy metals such as cadmium, lead, and mercury, often encountered in industrial settings or contaminated water and food supplies, interfere with mitochondrial function and catalyze the production of free radicals [7, 8].

Another major environmental contributor is radiation. Ultraviolet (UV) rays from excessive sun exposure and ionizing radiation from diagnostic tools or environmental sources can induce DNA damage directly, while also triggering ROS formation in surrounding tissues. Pesticides and other agricultural or industrial chemicals further exacerbate oxidative stress by disrupting redox-sensitive signaling pathways and impairing antioxidant defense mechanisms. Moreover, frequent exposure to heat, such as through hot tubs or saunas, and electromagnetic radiation from electronic devices, has been associated with oxidative damage in reproductive tissues, especially the testes, where temperature regulation is critical for sperm production [6, 9].

2.2 Lifestyle factors

Lifestyle choices also have a profound impact on the body's oxidative balance. Smoking introduces thousands of oxidants and free radicals into the body, overwhelming natural antioxidant systems and damaging sperm DNA, membranes, and proteins. Likewise, excessive alcohol consumption contributes to the production of toxic metabolites like acetaldehyde, which not only increase ROS generation but also impair antioxidant enzymes such as glutathione peroxidase. Poor dietary habits, particularly those lacking in fruits, vegetables, and essential micronutrients, further compromise the body's ability to neutralize oxidative agents. Diets high in saturated fats and processed foods are particularly harmful, promoting systemic inflammation and oxidative imbalance [10–13].

Physical activity can either support or disrupt redox homeostasis depending on intensity and duration. While moderate exercise is beneficial and supports antioxidant capacity, excessive or unregulated physical exertion without adequate recovery leads to increased mitochondrial respiration and, consequently, excess ROS production. Psychological stress also contributes significantly to oxidative stress. Chronic activation of the hypothalamic-pituitary-adrenal (HPA) axis elevates cortisol levels, alters metabolic function, and triggers the release of oxidative molecules. Additionally, inadequate sleep and unresolved psychological strain can suppress immune function and reduce antioxidant capacity. Recreational drug use and the chronic use of certain pharmaceuticals, such as chemotherapeutic agents, further increase oxidative burden by interfering with normal mitochondrial processes [14, 15].

Both environmental exposures and lifestyle behaviors can disrupt the delicate balance between ROS production and antioxidant defense, leading to oxidative stress.

This imbalance is especially detrimental to reproductive health, where oxidative damage has been closely linked to decreased sperm quality, DNA fragmentation, and reduced fertility potential. Addressing these factors through behavioral changes and protective interventions is essential for mitigating oxidative stress and supporting overall health [13, 16, 17].

3. Types of antioxidants and methods of administration and therapeutic potential

3.1 Types of antioxidants

Antioxidants are molecules that protect cells from oxidative stress by neutralizing free radicals, which are unstable compounds that can damage DNA, proteins, and lipids. These protective agents can be either naturally occurring or synthetically produced [18].

Natural antioxidants are commonly found in fruits, vegetables, nuts, and whole grains. Among the most well-known are vitamins such as vitamin C and vitamin E. Vitamin C is water-soluble and acts primarily in cellular fluids; it is abundant in citrus fruits, berries, and peppers. Vitamin E, on the other hand, is fat-soluble and protects cell membranes from lipid peroxidation. It is found in seeds, vegetable oils, and nuts [19, 20].

Minerals such as selenium and zinc also play critical antioxidant roles, though they do not act directly as antioxidants. Instead, they are cofactors for antioxidant enzymes. For instance, selenium is essential for the proper function of glutathione peroxidase, an enzyme that reduces harmful peroxides in cells.

In addition to these, polyphenols and flavonoids are important plant-based antioxidants. These compounds are found in richly colored foods such as berries, red wine, green tea, and dark chocolate. They often act by inhibiting the formation of free radicals and enhancing the activity of endogenous antioxidant enzymes [18, 20–22].

The human body also produces its own antioxidant defenses. These endogenous antioxidants include enzymes such as superoxide dismutase (SOD), catalase, and glutathione peroxidase, as well as small molecules such as glutathione and uric acid. These compounds work together to neutralize free radicals and maintain redox balance within cells [23].

On the other side, synthetic antioxidants are manufactured compounds used primarily in food preservation and industrial applications. Chemicals such as butylated hydroxytoluene (BHT) and butylated hydroxyanisole (BHA) are added to processed foods to prevent oxidation and spoilage. While effective, their safety in high or prolonged exposure is a topic of ongoing scientific debate [22, 24].

3.2 Methods of administration and therapeutic potential

Improving semen quality with antioxidants is a well-researched approach that targets one of the key causes of male infertility: oxidative stress.

To counteract the oxidative stress, antioxidants can be introduced into the body in a few effective ways, the most common being through oral supplementation [25].

Oral antioxidant therapy is widely used because it is non-invasive and easy to incorporate into daily life. Men who seek to improve their fertility are often advised to take supplements that include a blend of antioxidant compounds. These may contain vitamins, such as vitamin C and vitamin E, as well as minerals such as zinc and selenium, all of which support sperm health by protecting cells from free radical damage and aiding in DNA repair. Other compounds frequently included in these formulations are coenzyme Q10 and L-carnitine, both of which play a role in cellular energy production and are believed to enhance sperm motility. N-acetylcysteine, a precursor to glutathione, is also used to strengthen the body's own antioxidant defenses. These supplements are typically taken over a period of several months, aligning with the natural cycle of sperm development [26–28].

Alongside supplementation, diet is another important route for antioxidant intake. A nutrient-rich diet that emphasizes fruits, vegetables, nuts, seeds, and whole grains naturally provides the body with a wide variety of antioxidants, including flavonoids and carotenoids. Studies suggest that men who adopt dietary patterns high in these foods, such as the Mediterranean diet, often see improvements in sperm parameters, possibly due to the anti-inflammatory and antioxidant properties of the diet as a whole [25, 28, 29].

However, less common, intravenous administration of antioxidants has also been explored, particularly in medical contexts where high oxidative stress is present. In these cases, compounds such as vitamin C or glutathione are delivered directly into the bloodstream, offering immediate availability to tissues. However, this method is not typically used as a first-line treatment for infertility due to its invasive nature and the lack of large-scale evidence for its effectiveness in this specific application [30, 31].

The use of antioxidant supplementation in semen extenders is particularly relevant in the setting of assisted reproductive technologies (ART), most notably during sperm cryopreservation. This process is commonly used when men wish to preserve fertility, before undergoing medical treatments like chemotherapy, before a vasectomy, or as part of an *in vitro* fertilization procedure. While cryopreservation is effective, it poses significant challenges for sperm cells due to the physical and chemical stresses involved. These stresses, especially during the freezing and thawing stages, often result in oxidative damage, which can compromise sperm motility, membrane integrity, and DNA quality (**Table 1**) [32–34].

Sperm cells are highly sensitive to oxidative stress because of their limited natural antioxidant defenses and their membrane composition, which is rich in polyunsaturated fatty acids, particularly vulnerable to peroxidation. When semen is processed and stored at low temperatures, reactive oxygen species tend to accumulate. To reduce the extent of this damage, antioxidants can be introduced directly into the semen extender, the fluid that surrounds and protects sperm during storage. This strategy offers a localized and immediate form of protection, helping preserve functional sperm characteristics during and after thawing [23].

Research in this area has explored a range of antioxidant compounds that may be added to these extenders. Some are naturally occurring vitamins and enzymes with the protective roles, while others are synthetic or derived from plant sources. When used appropriately, they can improve key aspects of sperm quality, including motility and DNA stability, and may increase the success rates of reproductive treatments using frozen-thawed sperm [33, 35].

However, despite promising results in laboratory studies, the routine clinical use of antioxidant-enriched extenders in male fertility preservation is still somewhat limited. There are challenges in determining the most effective types and concentrations of antioxidants, as an imbalance can sometimes cause more harm than good. Excess antioxidants may disrupt the normal cellular signaling mechanisms or even act as pro-oxidants under certain conditions. Because of this, ongoing research continues to refine the formulations used and assess their real-world outcomes in human fertility treatments [34, 37].

Method of administration	Examples / compounds	Mechanism of action	Application /notes	References
Oral supplementation	Vitamin C (water soluble), vitamin E (fat-soluble), zinc, selenium, coenzyme Q10 L-carnitine, N-acetylcysteine	Neutralize free radicals, support DNA repair, enhance mitochondrial function and sperm motility, boost endogenous antioxidant enzymes	Widely used in male infertility treatments - Aligns with sperm development cycle (approx. 3 months)	[25–28]
Dietary intake	Fruits, vegetables, nuts, seeds, whole grains, flavonoids, carotenoids Mediterranean diet pattern	Natural antioxidant supply Anti-inflammatory properties Improve sperm parameters	Practical, long-term strategy, supports systemic health and fertility	[25, 28, 29]
Intravenous (IV) administration	Vitamin C glutathione	Rapid systemic availability, high dose antioxidant delivery	Used in high oxidative stress contexts, not common in standard infertility treatment due to invasiveness and limited evidence	[30, 31]
Antioxidant-enriched semen extenders	Vitamins (e.g., C, E), enzymes (e.g., SOD, catalase), plant derived or synthetic antioxidants	Direct protection of sperm during freezing/thawing—prevent lipid peroxidation and DNA damage	Used in cryopreservation (ART, IVF, chemo patients)—enhances post-thaw sperm quality and fertility potential	[23, 32–36]
Endogenous antioxidants *(produced by the body)*	Glutathione, uric acid, enzymes: SOD, catalase, glutathione peroxidase	Maintain cellular redox balance, work in synergy with dietary/supplemental antioxidants	Essential part of systemic antioxidant defense	[23]

Table 1.
Methods of antioxidant administration and their roles in male fertility.

Antioxidant supplementation in semen extenders represents a promising approach to reducing the oxidative stress associated with sperm cryopreservation. While the concept is well established in animal reproduction, its application in human fertility is still evolving, with careful attention being paid to optimizing safety and efficacy for clinical use (**Table 1**) [23, 36].

While multiple avenues exist for administering antioxidants to improve semen quality, oral supplementation and dietary intake remain the most practical and widely recommended methods. Their effectiveness is further enhanced when combined with lifestyle adjustments that reduce sources of oxidative damage.

4. Sociocultural or demographic differences in access to antioxidant-based interventions

Access to antioxidant-based interventions, whether through diet, supplements, or healthcare, varies widely across different social, cultural, and demographic groups.

These differences often reflect deeper inequalities in income, education, cultural norms, and healthcare systems, which can have real consequences for health, including issues related to oxidative stress and male fertility [38].

People with lower incomes, for example, may struggle to afford fresh fruits, vegetables, and other antioxidant rich foods. Instead, they may rely more heavily on cheaper, processed foods that lack essential nutrients. In contrast, individuals from higher-income backgrounds are more likely to afford a varied, nutrient-rich diet and have access to antioxidant supplements or specialized treatments [38].

Education also plays a key role. People who are more informed about health and nutrition are more likely to understand the benefits of antioxidants and how to include them in their diets. Meanwhile, those with limited health literacy might not be aware of the role antioxidants play in protecting the body from oxidative stress or supporting reproductive health [39].

Cultural beliefs and traditions can also shape how people view and use antioxidant therapies. In some cultures, people may prefer conventional medical treatments and be less open to dietary or supplement-based interventions. In others, especially where traditional medicine is widely practiced, there may be greater trust in natural or plant-based antioxidants. However, even in these cases, access to reliable and safe formulations may be limited [38].

Where someone lives also matters. People in rural or remote areas often have fewer options when it comes to buying fresh produce or getting advice from healthcare providers. Urban populations generally have better access to healthcare, nutrition education, and health-promoting services, which can make it easier for them to adopt antioxidant-rich diets or use supplements.

Lastly, the structure of the healthcare system itself can make a difference. In countries with strong public health programs, antioxidant-based care may be more widely available and affordable. But in places where healthcare is largely privatized or under resourced, these interventions might be considered extras available mostly to those who can pay out of pocket [39, 40].

Social and demographic factors have a major impact on who gets access to antioxidant-based support and who does not. To reduce these gaps, efforts need to focus on education, affordable nutrition, culturally appropriate healthcare, and policies that make antioxidant-rich foods and interventions more accessible to everyone.

5. Benefits and limitations of antioxidant use

5.1 Benefits

The idea of using antioxidants to improve health, especially in relation to oxidative stress and male fertility, has gained a lot of attention in recent years. While there is certainly evidence suggesting that antioxidants can be beneficial, the full picture is more nuanced, and there are important limitations to keep in mind when considering their use [41].

On the positive side, several clinical studies have shown that antioxidants can help reduce the damage caused by oxidative stress, which is known to affect sperm quality. Supplements such as vitamin C, vitamin E, selenium, zinc, and coenzyme Q10 have been linked to improvements in sperm motility, count, and overall function. Some research even suggests that antioxidant therapy can increase the chances of conception in couples facing male infertility. Some studies found that antioxidant supplements improved pregnancy and live birth rates in subfertility men, giving some weight to the idea that these treatments can be effective [42–44].

Antioxidants have also been studied outside the fertility space, in areas such as heart disease, neurodegenerative disorders, and diabetes. In some of these contexts, they appear to reduce inflammation or support mitochondrial function, which is encouraging [43].

That said, antioxidant therapy is far from a guaranteed fix. One of the biggest challenges in evaluating the evidence is how different the studies are from each other. They often vary in terms of the types of antioxidants used, how much people take, how long the treatments last, and the specific health conditions being targeted. This makes it hard to compare results or develop clear guidelines.

5.2 Limitations

While antioxidant therapy shows promise, particularly in areas such as male infertility and oxidative stress-related diseases, there are several important limitations and concerns that need to be acknowledged. These limitations often make it difficult to fully endorse widespread antioxidant use without careful consideration.

One of the major issues is the inconsistency in clinical outcomes. Although some studies report clear benefits, others show little to no improvement, and in some cases, even adverse effects. These conflicting results often stem from differences in study design. Clinical trials on antioxidants vary widely in terms of which substances are used, how much is administered, how long treatments last, and who the participants are. Without consistency across trials, it becomes difficult to draw firm conclusions or develop universal guidelines for use [45, 46].

Another limitation is the potential for harm when antioxidants are taken in excess. Although they are often marketed as harmless or even essential supplements, certain antioxidants can act as pro oxidants at high doses, meaning that instead of protecting cells, they may actually cause oxidative damage. For example, while vitamin E is commonly taken for its protective effects, some high-dose trials have shown it might increase the risk of prostate cancer or stroke. Similarly, beta-carotene, another well-known antioxidant, was found to increase the risk of lung cancer in smokers when taken in large amounts. These findings challenge the widespread belief that "more is better" when it comes to supplementation and highlight the importance of proper dosing [47].

There is also the issue of individual variability. The effectiveness of antioxidant therapy can differ significantly from person to person, depending on a range of factors including genetics, baseline antioxidant levels, diet, lifestyle, and overall health. Someone with a nutrient deficient diet might benefit from supplementation, while another person with adequate intake could experience no added benefit, or even harm. This variability complicates efforts to standardize treatment and calls for a more personalized approach rather than blanket recommendations [48, 49].

In addition, many antioxidants used in supplements do not always behave in the body the same way they do in controlled lab settings. Some compounds may not be well absorbed when taken orally, or they may be rapidly metabolized and cleared before having a meaningful effect. These points to a gap between laboratory findings and real world clinical effectiveness, further complicating their use.

Lastly, a broader concern is the lack of regulation and quality control in the supplement industry. In many countries, antioxidant supplements are sold over-the-counter with minimal oversight. This means that product quality, purity, and dosage can vary from brand to brand. Consumers may unknowingly take supplements that contain contaminants, incorrect doses, or misleading health claims. Without proper medical guidance, this increases the risk of both ineffectiveness and unintended health consequences [47].

While antioxidants have the potential to support health, their use comes with important caveats. The inconsistent clinical evidence, potential for harm at high doses, individual variability in response, and lack of standardization make it clear that antioxidant therapy should not be treated as a cure-all. Instead, these interventions are best used as part of a well-rounded, medically supervised approach to health, especially for conditions like male infertility where oxidative stress plays a known role. Further research, better regulation, and more personalized treatment strategies are all needed to unlock their full potential safely [49, 50].

6. Antioxidants, male reproductive aging, and public health: Implications for delayed fatherhood and fertility preservation

More men than ever are choosing to become fathers later in life. Whether it is because of career goals, financial stability, or personal reasons, this trend of delayed fatherhood is shaping new challenges for men's reproductive health. Unlike women, men do not have a strict biological "deadline" for fertility, but that does not mean their reproductive health stays the same as they age. In fact, aging can lead to declines in sperm quality, and antioxidants might hold some promise in helping men maintain fertility for longer but it is not a simple fix.

6.1 The role of antioxidants in age-related male fertility decline

As men get older, the cells in their bodies naturally face more stress, including something called oxidative stress. This happens when there is an imbalance between harmful molecules known as ROS and the body's ability to neutralize them. With advancing age, men experience a progressive increase in ROS production, particularly within the mitochondria of germ cells. This is often accompanied by a decline in the efficiency of antioxidant defense systems, such as the reduced activity of superoxide dismutase (SOD), catalase, and glutathione peroxidase (GPx). The imbalance between ROS generation and antioxidant capacity results in cumulative oxidative stress, which has been directly linked to decreased sperm motility, increased DNA fragmentation, and epigenetic instability in aging spermatozoa [51].

Additionally, oxidative stress affects testicular somatic cells and the hypothalamic-pituitary-gonadal (HPG) axis, contributing to lower testosterone levels and diminished spermatogenic output. Mitochondrial dysfunction and lipid peroxidation of the sperm plasma membrane further compromise sperm viability and fertilization capacity in older men.

Over time, this imbalance can damage sperm DNA, reduce sperm movement, and even lower sperm counts. All of these changes can make it harder to conceive naturally and increase the risk of health issues in children.

This is where antioxidants enter the picture. Antioxidants are substances that help neutralize ROS, protecting cells, including sperm, from damage. Vitamins like C and E, minerals such as selenium and zinc, and compounds like coenzyme Q10 have been studied for their ability to improve sperm health by reducing oxidative stress. Although antioxidants cannot stop aging altogether, they might help slow down some of the damage, giving men a better chance to have healthy sperm later in life [52].

It is important to remember, though, that antioxidants are not a magic bullet. They work best when combined with a healthy lifestyle, things like balanced nutrition, regular exercise, and avoiding smoking or excessive alcohol. Still, for men who are concerned about fertility and aging, antioxidants could be a useful piece of the puzzle.

6.2 Antioxidants and fertility preservation in the modern age

With more men thinking about having kids later, fertility preservation is becoming a hot topic. Sperm banking used to be something mainly recommended for men facing medical treatments like chemotherapy, but now many healthy men are considering it as a way to "freeze time" on their fertility.

Antioxidants may have a role here too. Some research suggests that taking antioxidants before sperm freezing can improve the quality of sperm after thawing, which is crucial for successful future use. Also, maintaining antioxidant levels through diet and lifestyle can help keep sperm healthier overall, making sperm banking more effective [2, 12].

For men planning ahead, antioxidant support alongside fertility preservation strategies offers a proactive approach, helping them protect their chances of becoming fathers even if they choose to wait.

6.3 Public health considerations and policy recommendations

From a bigger picture perspective, male fertility is an important public health issue that often gets overlooked. Around 15% of couples worldwide experience infertility, and male factors contribute to about half of these cases. Despite this, most public health messages focus on women's reproductive health, leaving men out of the conversation.

This needs to change. Educating men early starting in schools and continuing through healthcare providers, about how age, lifestyle, and things like oxidative stress affect fertility is crucial. When men understand these risks, they can make better choices about their health and family planning.

Access is another big piece of the puzzle. Not everyone has easy access to fresh fruits, vegetables, or supplements rich in antioxidants, especially in low-income or rural communities. Public health policies could help by subsidizing healthy foods, improving nutrition education, and making antioxidant-rich diets more affordable and accessible [2].

Healthcare systems also need to step up. Routine reproductive health check-ups for men, especially those over 35 or planning delayed fatherhood, should include advice on antioxidants, lifestyle changes, and fertility preservation options. This kind of proactive care could prevent many cases of infertility or reduce the need for expensive fertility treatments down the line.

Finally, there is the issue of supplements themselves. The market is flooded with antioxidant products that vary widely in quality and claims. Governments and regulators should tighten rules to ensure that supplements are safe, effective, and accurately labeled, so consumers are not misled or put at risk [14].

Antioxidants fit into a much bigger conversation about men's health, aging, and fertility in today's world. As fatherhood is delayed, men face challenges related to aging sperm and oxidative stress, but antioxidants offer a hopeful, if partial, tool to support reproductive health [16].

However, antioxidants work best as part of a broader, balanced approach, good nutrition, healthy habits, medical guidance, and supportive public policies. By combining these efforts, we can help men not only protect their fertility but also promote healthier families and communities in the end.

7. Emerging antioxidant therapies and advanced delivery systems: Innovations in combating oxidative stress and preserving male fertility

Recent biomedical advances are transforming the landscape of antioxidant therapy, particularly in the context of male infertility. Traditional antioxidant supplementation, though widely used, often falls short in efficacy due to poor targeting, bioavailability, and variability in individual oxidative stress responses. Innovations in both emerging antioxidant compounds and advanced delivery technologies, especially nanotechnology, are now offering new avenues to enhance treatment precision and outcomes. These developments are especially relevant in an era marked by delayed fatherhood, increased exposure to environmental stressors, and age-related fertility decline [1].

7.1 Targeted and potent antioxidants: Moving beyond traditional supplements

A growing body of research has introduced antioxidant compounds with improved specificity, potency, and cellular uptake, particularly those designed to target mitochondrial ROS production, which is central to sperm dysfunction.

Compounds such as Mitoquinone (MitoQ) and Plastoquinonyl-decyl-triphenylphosphonium (SkQ1) have been engineered to localize within mitochondria using lipophilic cations. By targeting the main site of ROS generation in sperm cells, these agents help restore mitochondrial function, enhance sperm motility, and reduce DNA fragmentation. Preclinical findings suggest their superior efficacy compared to conventional antioxidants [53].

Naturally derived antioxidants such as quercetin, resveratrol, and curcumin offer multifaceted protection by directly scavenging ROS and modulating pathways involved in inflammation, apoptosis, and mitochondrial biogenesis. Their epigenetic and anti-inflammatory effects make them particularly promising for long-term reproductive support [54].

Engineered molecules that mimic antioxidant enzymes (e.g., SOD mimetics or catalase analogues) exhibit catalytic activity and continuous ROS detoxification, offering sustained protection over time. These agents hold potential in chronic oxidative stress scenarios, especially for men with underlying metabolic disorders [18].

7.2 Personalized antioxidant strategies: One size does not fit all

As the understanding of oxidative stress deepens, it is clear that uniform supplementation strategies may be insufficient. The development of personalized antioxidant therapies, driven by biomarker data and individual susceptibility, is becoming an essential evolution in male infertility management.

Seminal ROS levels, DNA fragmentation indices, and antioxidant enzyme profiles (e.g., SOD, GPx) can guide the selection and dosing of antioxidants. Clinicians can use these biomarkers to tailor interventions, reducing the risk of overtreatment or ineffective therapy [14].

Polymorphisms in genes related to oxidative defense affect how individuals respond to antioxidant treatments. Emerging data suggest that combining genomic and epigenetic profiling may help identify at-risk patients and match them with targeted therapies [55].

Environmental exposures, smoking, diet, obesity, and chronic conditions like diabetes all influence oxidative burden. Comprehensive antioxidant strategies must integrate lifestyle counseling with personalized supplementation for maximum benefit (**Table 2**) [56].

7.3 Nanotechnology: Transforming antioxidant delivery

While potent antioxidants offer theoretical advantages, their clinical impact is often limited by physiological barriers such as the blood-testis barrier (BTB) and

Category	Type/example	Mechanism/features	Potential benefits	References
Emerging antioxidants	Mitochondria-targeted antioxidants e.g., MitoQ, SkQ1	Accumulate in mitochondria to neutralize ROS at the source	Improved sperm motility, mitochondrial health, DNA integrity	[53]
	Polyphenols/flavonoids, for example, quercetin, resveratrol, curcumin	ROS scavenging, anti-inflammatory, epigenetic modulation	Multilevel protection of sperm cells	[54]
	Synthetic antioxidants/ enzyme mimetics, for example, SOD mimetics	Mimic natural enzymes for sustained ROS detoxification	Enhanced intracellular protection, longer activity duration	[18]
Personalized therapeutic approaches	Biomarker-guided therapy	Use of oxidative stress markers to tailor therapy	Higher efficacy, minimized overtreatment	[14]
	Genetic/epigenetic profiling	Stratify patients based on antioxidant gene polymorphisms	Precision targeted treatments	[55]
	Lifestyle-integrated therapy	Combines antioxidant use with behavior and health modification	Improved long-term reproductive outcomes	[56]
Nanotechnology-based delivery	Nano-carriers e.g., liposomes, SLNs, polymeric NPs	Improve antioxidant solubility, stability, and release	Increased bioavailability and therapeutic concentration	[57]
	Targeted delivery to testes	Nanoparticles engineered to cross the blood-testis barrier (BTB)	Direct action on germ cells with minimal systemic side effects	[58, 59]
	Controlled/sustained release	Polymers degrade gradually, allowing slow, continuous antioxidant delivery	Maintains optimal ROS balance over time	[57]
	Co-delivery systems	Encapsulate multiple antioxidants or combo therapies in one carrier	Synergistic action and broader protection	[57, 59]

Table 2.
Emerging antioxidant therapies and advanced delivery systems.

issues of stability and solubility. Nanotechnology-based delivery systems are revolutionizing this space by offering enhanced bioavailability, targeted delivery, and controlled release.

Nanocarriers, including liposomes, polymeric nanoparticles, and solid lipid nanoparticles (SLNs), protect antioxidants from degradation in the gastrointestinal tract and systemic circulation. These vehicles allow for improved cellular uptake and prolonged systemic presence, enhancing the therapeutic potential [57, 58].

To reach germ cells, nanoparticles can be engineered to cross the BTB using receptor, mediated transport or cell, penetrating ligands. For instance, nanoparticles conjugated with folate or transferrin show selective uptake by Sertoli or germ cells, increasing antioxidant concentration exactly where it is needed [59].

Nanocarriers can be designed to release antioxidants gradually, maintaining steady-state concentrations in reproductive tissues. This sustained release approach minimizes ROS spikes while avoiding the pitfalls of high single-dose toxicity or underdosing [57].

Advanced nanocarriers can co-deliver multiple therapeutic agents. For example, encapsulating vitamin E with coenzyme Q10 in one nanoparticle can produce synergistic effects. Moreover, antioxidants can be delivered alongside anti-inflammatory or mitochondrial-targeted drugs to comprehensively address sperm dysfunction (**Table 2**) [59].

7.4 Challenges and future directions

Despite these promising innovations, there are barriers to clinical translation. Many of the studies remain preclinical or early phase trials, and challenges such as long term safety, large scale manufacturing, and regulatory approvals must be addressed. Moreover, standardized assays for oxidative stress and robust algorithms for personalized treatment remain in development.

In addition to these scientific and technical hurdles, important ethical considerations must be taken into account. One of the major concerns is the risk of over supplementation, which can lead to a condition known as reductive stress, an imbalance in the opposite direction of oxidative stress. This can disrupt normal cellular signaling, impair physiological redox reactions, and even contribute to mitochondrial dysfunction and infertility. While antioxidants are often marketed as universally beneficial, excessive or inappropriate use may have unintended consequences, particularly when used without medical supervision.

The introduction of advanced delivery systems, such as nanoparticles and mitochondria targeted compounds, raises further ethical and safety concerns. These include uncertainties regarding long term biocompatibility, potential toxicity, and accumulation of nanomaterials in tissues. As these technologies move closer to clinical application, it becomes essential to establish rigorous safety protocols and ensure transparent regulatory review. There is also a risk that such therapies could be misused or prematurely commercialized, particularly in unregulated or cosmetic fertility markets, before sufficient evidence of safety and efficacy is available.

Equity and access also represent key ethical dimensions. Advanced antioxidant therapies and personalized medicine approaches may initially be available only to those who can afford them, potentially exacerbating existing healthcare disparities in fertility treatment.

Nevertheless, the integration of nanotechnology, emerging antioxidants, and precision medicine is likely to reshape the future of male fertility care. Continued research, clinician education, and strong ethical oversight will be key to ensuring these promising therapies are both scientifically grounded, clinically effective, and equitably accessible.

8. Novel applications: Beyond conventional fertility treatments

While antioxidants have traditionally been used as dietary supplements to improve natural sperm quality by mitigating oxidative damage, emerging research has revealed their potential for novel applications that extend well beyond conventional fertility therapies. These innovative uses san ART, fertility preservation strategies, and integrative approaches combining antioxidants with cutting-edge biomedical interventions, opening new avenues for improving male reproductive outcomes.

8.1 Integration with ART

Assisted reproductive technologies such as in vitro fertilization (IVF) and intracytoplasmic sperm injection (ICSI) have revolutionized the treatment of male infertility, yet they introduce new oxidative challenges. The processes involved in sperm handling, including washing, centrifugation, and cryopreservation, often expose sperm to elevated levels of ROS, which can compromise sperm viability and DNA integrity [60]. To address this, antioxidants are increasingly incorporated into ART protocols. Supplementing sperm preparation media with antioxidants like vitamin E, glutathione, or melatonin has shown promise in reducing oxidative damage during sperm processing [61]. More recently, nano-encapsulated antioxidants have been tested to enhance protection by providing sustained and targeted ROS scavenging during critical sperm manipulation steps [60].

Moreover, antioxidant enriched cryoprotectants are being developed to improve the outcomes of sperm freezing and thawing. Cryopreservation is associated with increased ROS production, which damages membrane lipids and DNA, reducing post thaw sperm motility and fertilizing capacity [23]. Incorporation of antioxidants such as coenzyme Q10 and resveratrol into cryopreservation media has been demonstrated in animal models to improve post thaw sperm quality, suggesting translational benefits for human fertility preservation [1].

8.2 Fertility preservation in at risk populations

Beyond elective sperm banking for delayed fatherhood, antioxidant therapies are gaining traction in preserving fertility in men exposed to gonadotoxic stressors. These include cancer patients undergoing chemotherapy or radiotherapy, individuals exposed to environmental toxins or occupational hazards, and men with metabolic or inflammatory disorders associated with elevated oxidative stress [21]. Administering antioxidants prior to or alongside gonadotoxic treatments may mitigate ROS induced damage to spermatogenic cells, thereby preserving endogenous sperm production. Additionally, antioxidants may improve the quality of sperm cryopreserved for fertility preservation, enhancing the likelihood of successful conception post treatment [37, 61].

This protective strategy aligns with the broader concept of oncofertility, integrating reproductive health into cancer care. As survival rates improve, preserving quality of life, including fertility, is a growing priority, and antioxidant supplementation represents a low risk, potentially effective adjunct in this context [11].

8.3 Synergistic use with regenerative medicine and emerging technologies

The field of regenerative medicine offers exciting possibilities for treating male infertility, particularly in cases of severe testicular damage or azoospermia. Spermatogonial stem cell (SSC) transplantation and testicular tissue grafting are promising experimental therapies aiming to restore spermatogenesis. Antioxidants may play a crucial supportive role in these approaches by creating a protective microenvironment that enhances stem cell survival and function. Oxidative stress is a major cause of stem cell senescence and dysfunction; thus, antioxidant supplementation may improve the viability and proliferative capacity of SSCs both in vitro and after transplantation. Antioxidants could also be incorporated into scaffolds or biomaterials used for tissue engineering, ensuring sustained ROS protection during tissue regeneration [23, 59].

Furthermore, gene editing technologies such as CRISPR-Cas9 hold potential for correcting genetic causes of infertility. Since oxidative stress can influence gene expression and epigenetic modifications, antioxidant therapy may optimize the cellular milieu for gene editing procedures, improving efficacy and safety [62].

8.4 Emerging diagnostic and monitoring applications

Novel applications of antioxidants also extend into diagnostic realms. Biosensors and imaging agents incorporating antioxidant moieties are being developed to detect and quantify oxidative stress in real-time within reproductive tissues or seminal fluid. Such technologies could enable personalized antioxidant therapy by allowing clinicians to tailor treatments based on precise measurements of oxidative damage [23].

Theranostic nanoparticles, combining therapeutic and diagnostic functions, are under investigation to simultaneously deliver antioxidants and monitor their effects, thereby providing feedback for treatment optimization [63].

The expanding landscape of antioxidant applications reflects their versatile role in managing male reproductive health. From enhancing the safety and efficacy of assisted reproduction and fertility preservation to supporting regenerative therapies and enabling precision medicine, antioxidants are poised to become integral components of advanced fertility care. Continued research and clinical validation will be essential to translate these innovative approaches into routine practice, ultimately improving reproductive outcomes for a broad spectrum of men facing fertility challenges.

8.5 Challenges and future directions

Despite these exciting advances, several challenges remain. Translating nanotechnology, based antioxidants from bench to bedside requires extensive safety and efficacy testing to address potential toxicity, immunogenicity, and long term effects. Personalized antioxidant therapy demands integration of complex multi omics data into clinical workflows, necessitating robust bioinformatics tools and interdisciplinary collaboration. Regulatory frameworks must also evolve to keep pace with novel delivery platforms and therapeutic agents.

Emerging antioxidants, combined with cutting edge delivery systems and personalized medicine approaches, represent a promising evolution in managing oxidative stress related male infertility. These innovations have the potential to enhance treatment efficacy, reduce side effects, and ultimately improve reproductive outcomes, especially in the context of aging and environmental challenges. Continued research and clinical validation will be critical to realize their full potential and to integrate these technologies into standard fertility care.

9. Conclusions

The growing body of evidence clearly establishes oxidative stress as a key contributor to male infertility. Through its damaging effects on sperm DNA, membranes, and mitochondrial function, elevated levels of ROS compromise reproductive potential in both clinical and subclinical populations. Recognizing and addressing oxidative stress should become a cornerstone of male fertility assessments and treatment.

Antioxidants offer more than a reactive solution, they represent a proactive strategy for preserving male fertility across the lifespan. Their ability to restore redox balance, protect genetic integrity, and support mitochondrial health positions them as valuable agents in both therapeutic and preventive contexts. However, their effectiveness depends on dosage, bioavailability, and individual health status, necessitating careful, evidence based application.

As the field advances, it is becoming increasingly clear that a one-size-fits-all approach to antioxidant therapy may be suboptimal. Personalized strategies, guided by biomarkers of oxidative damage or genetic predisposition, are more likely to yield meaningful improvements in fertility outcomes. At the same time, innovations like nanotechnology and mitochondria targeted delivery systems hold promise for increasing efficacy and minimizing systemic side effects.

With trends toward delayed fatherhood, increased environmental exposures, and changing lifestyle factors, there is a pressing need to reframe male fertility as a long term health issue. Antioxidants can play a vital role in this new paradigm, not just in treating infertility but in preserving reproductive capacity over time. Public health strategies must evolve to include education, early screening, and access to evidence based interventions for all populations.

The clinical benefits of antioxidant therapy must be matched by public health and policy initiatives that ensure equitable access to treatment. Socioeconomic disparities, limited awareness, and fragmented healthcare services remain barriers to the widespread adoption of antioxidant based fertility preservation. Multidisciplinary collaboration among clinicians, researchers, and policymakers will be essential to translate scientific advancements into meaningful health outcomes.

Conflict of interest

The authors declare no conflict of interest.

DOI: http://dx.doi.org/10.5772/intechopen.1011991

Author details

Daniel Ionut Berean
Department of Reproduction, Faculty of Veterinary Medicine, University of Agricultural Sciences and Veterinary Medicine Cluj-Napoca, Cluj-Napoca, Romania

*Address all correspondence to: daniel.berean@usamvcluj.ro

References

[1] Rostamzadeh A, Anjamrooz SH, Rezaie MJ, Fathi F, Mohammadi M. Biological effects of magnetic resonance imaging on testis histology and seminiferous tubules morphometry. Oman Medical Journal. 2019;**34**(6): 544-552. DOI: 10.5001/omj.2019.98

[2] Barati E, Nikzad H, Karimian M. Oxidative stress and male infertility: Current knowledge of pathophysiology and role of antioxidant therapy in disease management. Cellular and Molecular Life Sciences. 2020;**77**(1):93-113. DOI: 10.1007/s00018-019-03253-8. Epub 2019 Aug 3

[3] Vahedi Raad M, Firouzabadi AM, Tofighi Niaki M, Henkel R, Fesahat F. The impact of mitochondrial impairments on sperm function and male fertility: A systematic review. Reproductive Biology and Endocrinology. 2024;**22**(1):83. DOI: 10.1186/s12958-024-01252-4

[4] Escada-Rebelo S, Cristo MI, Ramalho-Santos J, Amaral S. Mitochondria-targeted compounds to assess and improve human sperm function. Antioxidants & Redox Signaling. 2022;**37**(7-9):451-480. DOI: 10.1089/ars.2021.0238. Epub 2022 Mar 10

[5] Xu R, Zhong Y, Li R, Li Y, Zhong Z, Liu T, et al. Association between exposure to ambient air pollution and semen quality: A systematic review and meta-analysis. Science of the Total Environment. 2023;**870**:161892. DOI: 10.1016/j.scitotenv.2023.161892. Epub 2023 Jan 31

[6] Donkin I, Barrès R. Sperm epigenetics and influence of environmental factors. Molecular Metabolism. 2018;**14**:1-11. DOI: 10.1016/j.molmet.2018.02.006. Epub 2018 Feb 27

[7] Siddeek B, Mauduit C, Simeoni U, Benahmed M. Sperm epigenome as a marker of environmental exposure and lifestyle, at the origin of diseases inheritance. Mutation Research, Reviews in Mutation Research. 2018;**778**:38-44. DOI: 10.1016/j.mrrev.2018.09.001. Epub 2018 Sep 7

[8] Zhang F, Li H, Xu W, Song G, Wang Z, Mao X, et al. Sulfur dioxide may predominate in the adverse effects of ambient air pollutants on semen quality among the general population in Hefei, China. Science of the Total Environment. 2023;**867**:161472. DOI: 10.1016/j.scitotenv.2023.161472. Epub 2023 Jan 10

[9] Sun S, Zhao J, Cao W, Lu W, Zheng T, Zeng Q. Identifying critical exposure windows for ambient air pollution and semen quality in Chinese men. Environmental Research. 2020;**189**:109894. DOI: 10.1016/j.envres.2020.109894. Epub 2020 Jul 11

[10] Shi X, Chan CPS, Waters T, Chi L, Chan DYL, Li TC. Lifestyle and demographic factors associated with human semen quality and sperm function. Systems Biology in Reproductive Medicine. 2018;**64**(5):358-367. DOI: 10.1080/19396368.2018.1491074. Epub 2018 Jul 23

[11] Salas-Huetos A, James ER, Aston KI, Jenkins TG, Carrell DT. Diet and sperm quality: Nutrients, foods and dietary patterns. Reproductive Biology. 2019;**19**(3):219-224. DOI: 10.1016/j.repbio.2019.07.005. Epub 2019 Jul 30

[12] Szabó A, Váncsa S, Hegyi P, Váradi A, Forintos A, Filipov T, et al. Lifestyle-,

environmental-, and additional health factors associated with an increased sperm DNA fragmentation: A systematic review and meta-analysis. Reproductive Biology and Endocrinology. 2023;**21**(1):5. DOI: 10.1186/s12958-023-01054-0

[13] Nassan FL, Chavarro JE, Tanrikut C. Diet and men's fertility: Does diet affect sperm quality? Fertility and Sterility. 2018;**110**(4):570-577. DOI: 10.1016/j.fertnstert.2018.05.025

[14] Kesari KK, Agarwal A, Henkel R. Radiations and male fertility. Reproductive Biology and Endocrinology. 2018;**16**(1):118. DOI: 10.1186/s12958-018-0431-1

[15] Benatta M, Kettache R, Buchholz N, Trinchieri A. The impact of nutrition and lifestyle on male fertility. Archivio Italiano di Urologia, Andrologia. 2020;**92**(2). DOI: 10.4081/aiua.2020.2.121

[16] Rotimi DE, Singh SK. Implications of lifestyle factors on male reproductive health. JBRA Assisted Reproduction. 2024;**28**(2):320-330. DOI: 10.5935/1518-0557.20240007

[17] Jurewicz J, Radwan M, Sobala W, Ligocka D, Radwan P, Bochenek M, et al. Lifestyle and semen quality: Role of modifiable risk factors. Systems Biology in Reproductive Medicine. 2014;**60**(1):43-51. DOI: 10.3109/19396368.2013.840687. Epub 2013 Sep 30

[18] Neha K, Haider MR, Pathak A, Yar MS. Medicinal prospects of antioxidants: A review. European Journal of Medicinal Chemistry. 2019;**178**:687-704. DOI: 10.1016/j.ejmech.2019.06.010. Epub 2019 Jun 13

[19] Hęś M, Dziedzic K, Górecka D, Jędrusek-Golińska A, Gujska E. Aloe vera (L.) Webb.: Natural sources of antioxidants - A review. Plant Foods for Human Nutrition. 2019;**74**(3):255-265. DOI: 10.1007/s11130-019-00747-5

[20] Liu ZQ. Why natural antioxidants are readily recognized by biological systems? 3D architecture plays a role! Food Chemistry. 2022;**380**:132143. DOI: 10.1016/j.foodchem.2022.132143. Epub 2022 Jan 19

[21] He L, He T, Farrar S, Ji L, Liu T, Ma X. Antioxidants maintain cellular redox homeostasis by elimination of reactive oxygen species. Cellular Physiology and Biochemistry. 2017;**44**(2):532-553. DOI: 10.1159/000485089. Epub 2017 Nov 17

[22] Kostova I. Synthetic and natural coumarins as antioxidants. Mini Reviews in Medicinal Chemistry. 2006;**6**(4):365-374. DOI: 10.2174/138955706776361457

[23] Berean DI, Bogdan LM, Cimpean R. Advancements in understanding and enhancing antioxidant-mediated sperm cryopreservation in small ruminants: Challenges and perspectives. Antioxidants (Basel). 2024;**13**(6):624. DOI: 10.3390/antiox13060624

[24] Das P, Brahmachari G, Chatterjee K, Choudhuri T. Synthetic antioxidants from a natural source can overtake the oncogenic stress management system and activate the stress-sensitized death of KSHV-infected cancer cells. International Journal of Molecular Medicine. 2022;**50**(3):117. DOI: 10.3892/ijmm.2022.5173. Epub 2022 Jul 20

[25] Beaven EA, Colthorpe KL, Spiers JG, Chen HJ, Lavidis NA, Albrecht J. Oral administration of green plant-derived chemicals and antioxidants alleviates stress-induced cellular oxidative challenge. Journal of Basic and Clinical Physiology and Pharmacology.

2016;**27**(5):515-521. DOI: 10.1515/jbcpp-2016-0006

[26] Gharagozloo P, Aitken RJ. The role of sperm oxidative stress in male infertility and the significance of oral antioxidant therapy. Human Reproduction. 2011;**26**(7):1628-1640. DOI: 10.1093/humrep/der132. Epub 2011 May 5

[27] Kumar GG, Kilari EK, Nelli G, Salleh NB. Oral administration of Turnera diffusa willd. ex Schult. extract ameliorates steroidogenesis and spermatogenesis impairment in the testes of rats with type-2 diabetes mellitus. Journal of Ethnopharmacology. 2023;**314**:116638. DOI: 10.1016/j.jep.2023.116638. Epub 2023 May 13

[28] Imamovic Kumalic S, Pinter B. Review of clinical trials on effects of oral antioxidants on basic semen and other parameters in idiopathic oligoasthenoteratozoospermia. BioMed Research International. 2014;**2014**:426951. DOI: 10.1155/2014/426951. Epub 2014 Mar 31

[29] Akmal M, Qadri JQ, Al-Waili NS, Thangal S, Haq A, Saloom KY. Improvement in human semen quality after oral supplementation of vitamin C. Journal of Medicinal Food. 2006;**9**(3):440-442. DOI: 10.1089/jmf.2006.9.440

[30] Greco E, Romano S, Iacobelli M, Ferrero S, Baroni E, Minasi MG, et al. ICSI in cases of sperm DNA damage: Beneficial effect of oral antioxidant treatment. Human Reproduction. 2005;**20**(9):2590-2594. DOI: 10.1093/humrep/dei091. Epub 2005 Jun 2

[31] Crosta F, Stefani A, Melani F, Fabrizzi P, Nizzardo A, Grassi D, et al. Improvement of executive function after short-term administration of an antioxidants mix containing bacopa, lycopene, astaxanthin and vitamin B12: The BLAtwelve study. Nutrients. 2020;**13**(1):56. DOI: 10.3390/nu13010056

[32] Hameed N, Akhter S, Souza-Fabjan JMG, Zubair M, Irfan-Ur-Rehman Khan M. Effects of different extenders, storage temperatures, and antioxidant supplementation on chilled semen quality: A review. Tropical Animal Health and Production. 2024;**56**(2):85. DOI: 10.1007/s11250-024-03930-2

[33] Nekoonam S, Nashtaei MS, Naji M, Zangi BM, Amidi F. Effect of Trolox on sperm quality in normozospermia and oligozospermia during cryopreservation. Cryobiology. 2016;**72**(2):106-111. DOI: 10.1016/j.cryobiol.2016.02.008. Epub 2016 Mar 2

[34] Ezzati M, Shanehbandi D, Hamdi K, Rahbar S, Pashaiasl M. Influence of cryopreservation on structure and function of mammalian spermatozoa: An overview. Cell and Tissue Banking. 2020;**21**(1):1-15. DOI: 10.1007/s10561-019-09797-0. Epub 2019 Dec 3

[35] Amidi F, Pazhohan A, Shabani Nashtaei M, Khodarahmian M, Nekoonam S. The role of antioxidants in sperm freezing: A review. Cell and Tissue Banking. 2016;**17**(4):745-756. DOI: 10.1007/s10561-016-9566-5. Epub 2016 Jun 24

[36] Huang C, Tang YL, Hu JL, Zhou WJ, Huang ZH, Luo XF, et al. Update on techniques for cryopreservation of human spermatozoa. Asian Journal of Andrology. 2022;**24**(6):563-569. DOI: 10.4103/aja20229

[37] Zhang X, Lu X, Li J, Xia Q, Gao J, Wu B. Mito-tempo alleviates cryodamage by regulating intracellular oxidative metabolism in spermatozoa from asthenozoospermic patients. Cryobiology. 2019;**91**:18-22.

DOI: 10.1016/j.cryobiol.2019.11.005. Epub 2019 Nov 14

[38] Lansford JE. Annual research review: Cross-cultural similarities and differences in parenting. Journal of Child Psychology and Psychiatry. 2022;**63**(4):466-479. DOI: 10.1111/jcpp.13539. Epub 2021 Nov 11

[39] Gonzalez-Tapia G, Lazzaro-Salazar M. Medical empathy in the physician-patient relationship: A review from a cultural perspective. Revista Médica de Chile. 2023;**151**(9):1233-1240. DOI: 10.4067/s0034-98872023000901233

[40] Ma X, Tamir M, Miyamoto Y. A socio-cultural instrumental approach to emotion regulation: Culture and the regulation of positive emotions. Emotion. 2018;**18**(1):138-152. DOI: 10.1037/emo0000315. Epub 2017 Apr 17

[41] Qian C, Meng Q, Lu J, Zhang L, Li H, Huang B. Human amnion mesenchymal stem cells restore spermatogenesis in mice with busulfan-induced testis toxicity by inhibiting apoptosis and oxidative stress. Stem Cell Research & Therapy. 2020;**11**(1):290. DOI: 10.1186/s13287-020-01803-7

[42] Alqawasmeh OA, Zhao M, Chan CP, Leung MB, Chow KC, Agarwal N, et al. Green tea extract as a cryoprotectant additive to preserve the motility and DNA integrity of human spermatozoa. Asian Journal of Andrology. 2021;**23**(2):150-156. DOI: 10.4103/aja.aja_58_20

[43] Kalthur G, Salian SR, Keyvanifard F, Sreedharan S, Thomas JS, Kumar P, et al. Supplementation of biotin to sperm preparation medium increases the motility and longevity in cryopreserved human spermatozoa. Journal of Assisted Reproduction and Genetics. 2012;**29**(7):631-635. DOI: 10.1007/s10815-012-9760-8. Epub 2012 Apr 21

[44] Brennan AP, Holden CA. Pentoxifylline-supplemented cryoprotectant improves human sperm motility after cryopreservation. Human Reproduction. 1995;**10**(9):2308-2312. DOI: 10.1093/oxfordjournals.humrep.a136291

[45] Santonastaso M, Mottola F, Iovine C, Colacurci N, Rocco L. Protective effects of curcumin on the outcome of cryopreservation in human sperm. Reproductive Sciences. 2021;**28**(10):2895-2905. DOI: 10.1007/s43032-021-00572-9. Epub 2021 Apr 16

[46] Si W, Benson JD, Men H, Critser JK. Osmotic tolerance limits and effects of cryoprotectants on the motility, plasma membrane integrity and acrosomal integrity of rat sperm. Cryobiology. 2006;**53**(3):336-348. DOI: 10.1016/j.cryobiol.2006.09.001. Epub 2006 Nov 3

[47] Forman HJ, Zhang H. Targeting oxidative stress in disease: Promise and limitations of antioxidant therapy. Nature Reviews. Drug Discovery. 2021;**20**(9):689-709. DOI: 10.1038/s41573-021-00233-1. Epub 2021 Jun 30. Erratum in: Nat Rev Drug Discov. 2021;20(8):652. doi: 10.1038/s41573-021-00267-5

[48] Steiner AZ, Hansen KR, Barnhart KT, Cedars MI, Legro RS, Diamond MP, et al. Reproductive medicine network. The effect of antioxidants on male factor infertility: The males, antioxidants, and infertility (MOXI) randomized clinical trial. Fertility and Sterility. 2020;**113**(3):552-560.e3. DOI: 10.1016/j.fertnstert.2019.11.008. Epub 2020 Feb 25

[49] Montero AJ, Jassem J. Cellular redox pathways as a therapeutic target in the treatment of cancer. Drugs.

2011;**71**(11):1385-1396. DOI: 10.2165/11592590-000000000-00000

[50] Sies H, Jones DP. Reactive oxygen species (ROS) as pleiotropic physiological signalling agents. Nature Reviews Molecular Cell Biology. 2020;**21**(7):363-383. DOI: 10.1038/s41580-020-0230-3. Epub 2020 Mar 30

[51] Sharma R, Biedenharn KR, Fedor JM, Agarwal A. Lifestyle factors and reproductive health: Taking control of your fertility. Reproductive Biology and Endocrinology. 2013;**11**:66. DOI: 10.1186/1477-7827-11-66

[52] Fraga CG, Motchnik PA, Wyrobek AJ, Rempel DM, Ames BN. Smoking and low antioxidant levels increase oxidative damage to sperm DNA. Mutation Research. 1996;**351**(2):199-203. DOI: 10.1016/0027-5107(95)00251-0

[53] Murphy MP, Holmgren A, Larsson NG, Halliwell B, Chang CJ, Kalyanaraman B, et al. Unraveling the biological roles of reactive oxygen species. Cell Metabolism. 2011;**13**(4):361-366. DOI: 10.1016/j.cmet.2011.03.010

[54] Aitken RJ. Impact of oxidative stress on male and female germ cells: Implications for fertility. Reproduction. 2020;**159**(4):R189-R201. DOI: 10.1530/REP-19-0452

[55] Gunes S, Esteves SC. Role of genetics and epigenetics in male infertility. Andrologia. 2021;**53**(1):e13586. DOI: 10.1111/and.13586. Epub 2020 Apr 21

[56] Esteves SC, Santi D, Simoni M. An update on clinical and surgical interventions to reduce sperm DNA fragmentation in infertile men. Andrology. 2020;**8**(1):53-81. DOI: 10.1111/andr.12724. Epub 2019 Dec 9

[57] Taouzinet L, Fatmi S, Lahiani-SkibaM, SkibaM, Iguer-OuadaM. Encapsulation nanotechnology in sperm cryopreservation: Systems preparation methods and antioxidants enhanced delivery. Cryo Letters. 2021;**42**(1):1-12

[58] Mili B, Chutia T, Buragohain L, Palanisammi A, Kumaresan A. Liquid storage of boar semen: Current approaches to reducing sperm damage using antioxidants and nanotechnology. Animal Reproduction Science. 2025;**278**:107871. DOI: 10.1016/j.anireprosci.2025.107871. Epub 2025 May 23

[59] Zandiyeh S, Kalantari H, Fakhri A, Nikkhah M, Janani BJ, Sabbaghian M. A review of recent developments in the application of nanostructures for sperm cryopreservation. Cryobiology. 2024;**115**:104890. DOI: 10.1016/j.cryobiol.2024.104890. Epub 2024 Apr 3

[60] Agarwal A, Durairajanayagam D, du Plessis SS. Utility of antioxidants during assisted reproductive techniques: An evidence based review. Reproductive Biology and Endocrinology. 2014;**12**:112. DOI: 10.1186/1477-7827-12-112

[61] Ribas-Maynou J, Yeste M. Oxidative stress in male infertility: Causes, effects in assisted reproductive techniques, and protective support of antioxidants. Biology (Basel). 2020;**9**(4):77. DOI: 10.3390/biology9040077

[62] Creta M, Arcaniolo D, Celentano G, Napolitano L, La Rocca R, Capece M, et al. Toxicity of antioxidant supplements in patients with male factor infertility: A systematic review and meta-analysis of randomized controlled trials. Antioxidants (Basel). 2021;**11**(1):89. DOI: 10.3390/antiox11010089

[63] Takalani NB, Monageng EM, Mohlala K, Monsees TK, Henkel R, Opuwari CS. Role of oxidative stress in male infertility. Reproduction and Fertility. 2023;**4**(3):e230024. DOI: 10.1530/RAF-23-0024

Section 2

Clinical Management and Therapeutic Interventions

Chapter 3

Urological Congenitalism, Reconstruction and Neuro-Urological Male Patients: Reproductive Health and Fertility Challenges and Their Contemporary Management

Talal A. Alenezi, Abdulrahman Almazeedi, Maryam Albuloushi, Ali Almoumen, Naser Al-Soudan Al-Anazi, Abdullatif E. Al-Terki, Tariq F. Al-Shaiji and Said M. Yaiesh

Abstract

Male patients with congenital urogenital anomalies and neuro-urological conditions represent a unique and underrecognized population at risk for infertility and sexual dysfunction. This chapter aims to review the embryological and developmental basis of these conditions and to clarify their direct effects on spermatogenesis, hormonal regulation, and sperm transport. We provide a detailed discussion of common anomalies—including bladder exstrophy, prune belly syndrome, cryptorchidism, and spinal dysraphism—as well as acquired neuro-urological disorders, such as multiple sclerosis, spinal cord injury, and cerebrovascular accident, highlighting their impact on reproductive health and quality of life. Key findings demonstrate that both congenital and neurogenic conditions disrupt male fertility through structural anomalies, impaired testicular development, endocrine dysfunction, and ejaculatory disorders. Contemporary management strategies—ranging from early orchiopexy, reconstructive and substitution phalloplasty, penile prostheses, and urinary tract reconstruction, to assisted reproductive technologies (ART) and sperm retrieval—can mitigate these challenges. Multidisciplinary care, involving functional and reproductive urology, endocrinology, neurology, and psychology, is shown to optimize fertility outcomes. Additionally, models of transitional urology illustrate how proactive fertility counseling and early intervention improve long-term reproductive prospects. In conclusion, congenitalism and neuro-urological disease exert profound effects on male reproductive health that extend beyond childhood survival into adulthood and family planning. Advances in surgical reconstruction, ART, and multidisciplinary care are improving outcomes; yet, long-term follow-up and fertility-preservation strategies remain critical. Future directions—including stem-cell therapy, neuromodulation, and AI-supported management—offer promise in addressing the unmet needs of this vulnerable population.

Keywords: neuro-urology, congenitalism, fertility, reconstruction, assisted reproduction

1. Introduction

Congenital anomalies of the kidney and urinary tract (CAKUT) account for 1% of all live births [1]. Along with external genital anomalies, CAKUT shares a common embryologic origin; thus, patients with CAKUT may suffer from infertility and sexual dysfunction [2]. These anomalies represent a significant challenge for any parent. The early-life challenges are related to the survival of their child and the quality of life (QoL) of the child and parents alike. The survival of such a group of patients has increased over the past years as the medical field has advanced. As the child grows to be socially independent, the challenges become different, as sexuality and reproductive function become a major concern [3]. As our understanding deepens of the relationship between male-factor infertility, which represents up to 50% of the causality in infertile couples, clearer connections are identified with male genitourinary congenitalism and management options [2].

Infertility and sexual dysfunction can also be of neurogenic origin. Multiple sclerosis (MS) carries a significant impact on fertility, sexuality, and quality of life [4]. An estimated 47–75% of males diagnosed with multiple sclerosis suffer from sexual dysfunction and lower testosterone production [5]. On the other hand, spinal cord injury (SCI) patients commonly suffer from sexual dysfunction, and 26% of patients prioritize the regain of sexual function [6]. The prevalence of post-stroke sexual dysfunction ranges between 20 and 75%. Low serum testosterone levels, infertility, and sexual dysfunction are common in this special population, which can negatively impact quality of life [7]. In this chapter, we aim to discuss these special populations with congenital urogenital anomalies and neurogenic diseases and their impacts on the sexual health and reproductive function of affected males.

1.1 Embryology of the urinary tract

Pronephros, mesonephros, and metanephros are the key structures in the development of the genitourinary tract. The intermediate mesoderm is the origin of these structures. The pronephros is a transient structure that regresses completely by the fifth week of gestation. The mesonephros differentiates into mesonephric tubules and mesonephric ducts, which form the epididymis, vas deferens, and seminal vesicles. In association with the urogenital sinus, they form the bladder and urethra. Also, its outgrowth forms the upper urinary tract, except for the nephron itself, which is formed by the metanephros. The kidney matures by 10 weeks of gestation, and its normal location is between spinal levels T10 and L3. Meanwhile, starting from the fourth gestational week, the cloaca divides into the urogenital sinus anteriorly and rectum posteriorly. Then, the urogenital sinus divides into three parts: the vesical part, which gives most of the bladder and is continuous with its allantois, the pelvic part, which gives the female

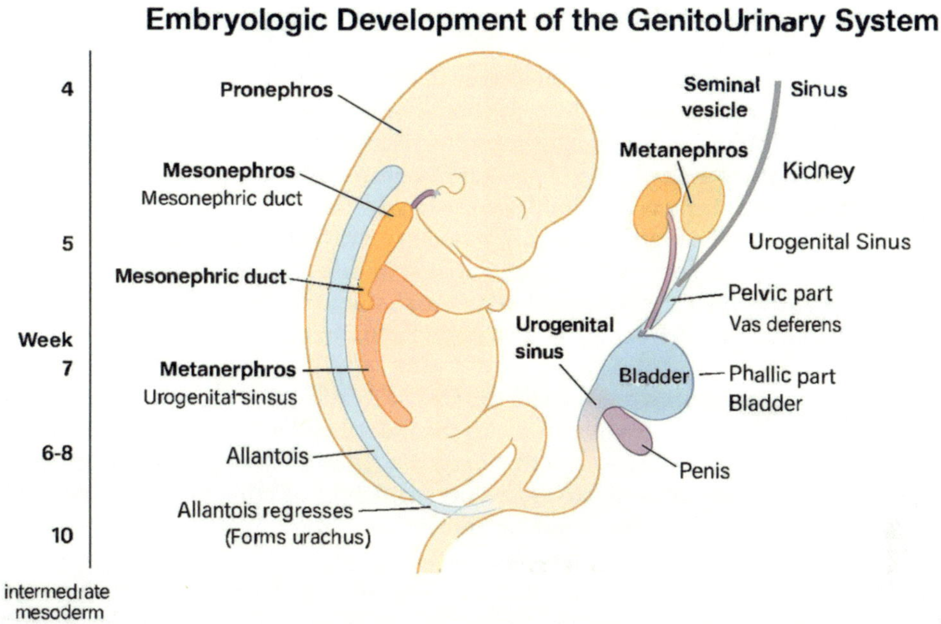

Figure 1.
Embryologic development of the genitourinary system – A snapshot.

urethra and the male prostatic urethra, and the phallic part, which gives the clitoris in females and the penis in males.

The allantois, which is responsible embryologically for gas exchange and waste elimination, also plays a role in umbilical cord formation. Later, by the sixth to eighth weeks of gestation, regression of the allantois occurs, and the intra-abdominal segment will form the urachus, which becomes the median umbilical ligament connecting the bladder dome to the anterior abdominal wall. The sex-determining-region Y (SRY) gene promotes secretion of the testis-determining factor, which initiates the formation of the testis and differentiation of Leydig and Sertoli cells. The testes develop from the intermediate mesoderm and initially form in the abdomen, then descend into the scrotum due to abdominal growth and the migratory action of the gubernaculum (**Figure 1**) [8, 9].

1.2 Generalized outlook on male reproductive health

Congenital anomalies of the kidney and urinary tract (CAKUT) encompass a spectrum of disorders that arise from disruptions in the embryological development of the intermediate mesoderm. This same embryologic layer also gives rise to components of the male reproductive tract, specifically *via* the mesonephric (Wolffian) duct. Consequently, the close anatomical and developmental association between the urinary and reproductive systems in the male means that CAKUT has not only renal consequences but also direct implications on spermatogenesis, sperm transport, and hormonal regulation. These effects are often underrecognized and may manifest later in life as unexplained subfertility or sexual dysfunction [2].

The earliest impact of CAKUT on the male reproductive system occurs during mesonephric duct development, which gives rise to the epididymis, vas deferens, seminal vesicles, and ejaculatory ducts. Anomalies in this developmental sequence can result in partial or complete agenesis of these structures [9]. For instance, congenital unilateral absence of the vas deferens (CUAVD), often found in conjunction with ipsilateral renal agenesis, reflects failure of mesonephric duct elongation and differentiation. Similarly, Zinner syndrome—a triad of renal agenesis, seminal vesicle cysts, and ejaculatory duct obstruction—represents a classic example where both urinary and reproductive tracts are simultaneously affected due to a shared mesonephric origin. Patients with these anomalies often present with infertility despite preserved spermatogenesis, due to obstructive azoospermia or defective ejaculatory function. Imaging modalities such as transrectal ultrasound and magnetic resonance imaging (MRI), in conjunction with semen analysis and hormonal evaluation, are essential for diagnosis and counseling [10, 11].

Beyond structural ductal abnormalities, CAKUT can exert a significant impact on spermatogenesis through both intrinsic and secondary mechanisms. CAKUT exerts multifaceted effects on male fertility that extend beyond structural abnormalities. For instance, posterior urethral valves and ureteropelvic junction obstruction cause recurrent urinary tract infections and chronic inflammation, which can impair epididymal function and seminal plasma composition, leading to reduced motility and DNA fragmentation in sperm. Clinical studies demonstrate that men with a history of posterior urethral valves are at significantly higher risk of subfertility, with paternity rates ranging between 40 and 60% compared to >85% in matched controls [2, 10–11].

Prune belly syndrome provides a particularly illustrative example: in a recent scoping review, over 75% of men were azoospermic, and only 2.7% demonstrated normal spermatogenesis on testicular histology. Even in cases with successful sperm retrieval, ART was required to achieve pregnancy. Similarly, bladder exstrophy-epispadias complex (BEEC) has been associated with erectile dysfunction in up to 63% of patients and abnormal ejaculation in 41%, contributing to low rates of spontaneous conception [11].

Additionally, in such syndromic variants like prune belly syndrome or severe posterior urethral valves, testicular descent is often impaired due to abdominal wall hypoplasia, increased intra-abdominal pressure, or abnormal gubernacular development [12]. Bilateral undescended testes, which occur in a significant majority of prune belly cases, contribute to abnormal thermal regulation of the testis and progressive germ cell loss [13]. Histologic studies in this population demonstrate a range of testicular dysgenesis patterns, including absent spermatogonia, hyalinization of seminiferous tubules, and Sertoli cell-only syndrome in up to half of patients. Even among those with descended testes or timely orchiopexy, early intrauterine injury to the testicular architecture may lead to impaired germ cell maturation and reduced fertility potential later in life [12, 13].

Moreover, longstanding upper and lower tract obstruction, which can occur in entities such as ureteropelvic junction obstruction or posterior urethral valves, may lead to repeated urinary tract infections and inflammation of the genitourinary tract. This chronic inflammatory state has been associated with oxidative stress, increased leukocytospermia, and damage to the epididymal or prostatic ducts. Over time, these effects can impair sperm motility, DNA integrity, and the composition of seminal plasma, all of which are essential for natural fertility. In some cases, scarring or stenosis of the ejaculatory ducts may occur, resulting in low-volume, acidic, and fructose-negative ejaculate—hallmarks of distal ejaculatory duct obstruction [14, 15].

Hormonal dysregulation is another underappreciated pathway by which CAKUT impacts male fertility. In patients with bilateral renal dysplasia or early-onset chronic kidney disease (CKD), disruption of the hypothalamic-pituitary-gonadal (HPG) axis is common. Uremia and metabolic acidosis impair the pulsatile secretion of gonadotropin-releasing hormone (GnRH), which leads to blunted luteinizing hormone (LH) and follicle-stimulating hormone (FSH) release and, ultimately, reduced intratesticular testosterone. This state of hypogonadotropic hypogonadism can manifest as diminished libido, erectile dysfunction, and impaired spermatogenesis [16]. In prepubertal and adolescent males with CKD due to CAKUT, delayed puberty or incomplete virilization may also occur. Elevated prolactin levels, seen frequently in CKD, further suppress GnRH secretion, compounding the endocrine dysfunction. Hormonal assays in these patients often reveal low testosterone, low or inappropriately normal gonadotropins, and reduced serum inhibin B—a surrogate marker of Sertoli cell activity and spermatogenic potential [17, 18].

It is also important to note that not all testicular abnormalities in CAKUT are secondary to cryptorchidism or obstruction. Some evidence suggests that intrinsic testicular dysgenesis may occur in certain syndromic CAKUT forms due to underlying genetic or epigenetic aberrations. For instance, patients with 17q12 microdeletion syndrome—associated with renal cystic dysplasia and maturity-onset diabetes of the young (MODY5)—may have concurrent gonadal anomalies due to transcription factor mutations that affect urogenital ridge development. These emerging data support the notion that the testes themselves may be developmentally impaired in some CAKUT patients, independent of their ductal or renal manifestations [19, 20].

By systematically addressing structural, hormonal, and inflammatory pathways, clinicians can better identify which CAKUT subtypes carry the highest fertility risk and tailor interventions accordingly. Given the multifaceted impact of CAKUT on the male reproductive axis, a comprehensive and proactive approach is warranted. Assessment should not be limited to imaging and renal function alone but must include endocrine profiling, semen analysis, and ultrasonographic evaluation of the reproductive tract. Early identification of abnormalities enables timely interventions, such as hormonal therapy, testicular sperm extraction (TESE), or referral for ART. In adolescents with known CAKUT, counseling regarding future fertility and potential preservation strategies—such as sperm cryopreservation in those undergoing reconstructive surgery or at risk of progressive renal disease—should be incorporated into routine care. Furthermore, the psychological implications of infertility or sexual dysfunction must not be overlooked and are best addressed within a multidisciplinary framework that includes reproductive urologists, endocrinologists, and mental-health professionals.

Thus, the impact of CAKUT on male reproductive health extends well beyond mechanical anomalies. Disruptions in spermatogenesis, sperm transport, and hormonal regulation often coexist and may not be clinically evident until adulthood. A structured, multidisciplinary approach with longitudinal surveillance is essential to preserve fertility and optimize quality of life in this growing patient population.

1.3 Specific anomalies of the upper urinary tract

The anomalies of the kidneys commonly manifest as unilateral or bilateral renal agenesis. Unilateral renal agenesis has an incidence of 1 in 1100 births, is more common in boys, and affects the left side more than the right side. Patients can be asymptomatic or may present with primary infertility, as it is associated with Wolffian duct anomalies such as Zinner syndrome or absence of the vas deferens, both of which will be discussed later in this chapter [21].

1.3.1 Horseshoe kidney

Horseshoe kidney is one of the most common anomalies of the urinary system and affects 0.25% of the general population, with a male-to-female ratio of 2:1. In 90% of cases, an isthmus typically connects the lower poles, while in a minority of cases, it connects the upper poles. In about 70% of the cases, the position of the kidney will be on the left lateral side. Patients are mostly asymptomatic, although in childhood, they may present with abdominal pain [22]. Horseshoe kidneys result in altered anatomical relationships within the retroperitoneum. This abnormal positioning can predispose individuals to compression of the left renal vein, a condition known as nutcracker syndrome [22].

1.3.1.1 Nutcracker syndrome

Nutcracker syndrome is caused by entrapment of the left renal vein between the aorta and the superior mesenteric artery (SMA), leading to increased resistance in the vein, which in turn can impair drainage of the left gonadal vein, ultimately resulting in the development of left varicoceles [23]. Patients may present with symptoms such as testicular or abdominal pain, while additional findings like oligoasthenospermia may be observed. All the aforementioned clinical features indicate the need for surgical intervention [22].

The recommended treatment for nutcracker syndrome in younger patients under 18 years of age and those who are underweight includes weight gain, ACE inhibitors, and aspirin. Surgical options are laparoscopic renal vein grafting with renal vein stenting or laparoscopic third extravascular stent placement. Another promising approach involves microvascular Doppler-assisted microsurgical left spermatic inferior epigastric vein anastomosis with microscopic varicocele ligation. The reasons to choose the inferior epigastric vein are easy accessibility during surgery, suitable caliber of the vein, and reduced risk of turbulent flow. However, data on this approach is limited, and further studies with long-term follow-up are needed [22].

1.3.2 Autosomal dominant polycystic kidney disease (ADPCKD)

ADPCKD is defined as multiple enlarged cysts in both kidneys along with multiple extrarenal manifestations, such as seminal vesicle, epididymal, liver, and pancreatic cysts, as well as berry aneurysms in the brain. It is an inherited disorder caused by mutations in the PKD1 and PKD2 genes, which are responsible for 85 and 15% of cases, respectively [24].

In both ADPKD and unilateral renal agenesis, infertility is commonly attributed to ejaculatory duct obstruction. Approximately 60% of patients with seminal vesicle cysts experience obstruction of the ejaculatory duct, leading to ejaculatory failure. Azoospermia is frequently observed in these cases [24]. A thorough history aids in forming a differential diagnosis, and a physical examination can identify the absence of the vas deferens. Seminal analysis is crucial to differentiate complete from partial ejaculatory duct obstruction. Imaging modalities used to confirm the diagnosis include vasography, transrectal ultrasound, seminal vesiculography, and MRI [25].

The management of ejaculatory duct obstruction will be discussed later, along with anomalies of the vas deferens and the ejaculatory duct.

1.4 Specific anomalies of the lower urinary tract

1.4.1 Bladder agenesis

Bladder agenesis is a rare congenital anomaly characterized by the absence of the urinary bladder. The available literature on the etiology of bladder agenesis and its associated anomalies is limited, thus explaining the pathophysiology of the disease is difficult [26]. The defect can be secondary to an atrophied vesical part of the urogenital sinus and defective fusion of the mesonephric duct and ureters into the bladder [27]. The immediate concern for patients with bladder agenesis is urinary drainage, as it is the most important determinant of compatibility with life [28].

In a systematic review conducted by Yahya et al., 65 bladder agenesis subjects were identified, 19 of whom were males. Associated anomalies were reported as cardiac, vascular, and musculo-skeletal. Associated urogenital anomalies were identified in 90% of subjects and included absent phallus, penoscrotal transposition, undescended testes, and underdeveloped scrotum. The mortality rate in male patients reached 74%. Eight out of the 19 patients had an absent phallus, and one patient had a small phallus. All identified cases passed away shortly after birth. Another reported case was of a 60-year-old male who presented with incontinence; interestingly, he had normal sexual function [29].

1.4.2 Bladder exstrophy-epispadias complex (BEEC)

BEEC is a spectrum of malformations that varies in presentation from simple epispadias to multisystemic defects [30]. The incidence of BEEC is 2.4 in 100,000 live births, with a male-to-female ratio of 2:1 [31]. Distal epispadias is the least severe form of the spectrum, whereas cloacal exstrophy is the most severe form. Associated genitourinary, gastrointestinal, and musculoskeletal anomalies are common. Surgical reconstruction of bladder exstrophy aims to achieve continence and to preserve sexual function.

1.4.2.1 Embryology and pathophysiology

Due to the failure of mesenchymal cells migration during the fourth gestational week, resulting in widening of the pubic symphysis, bladder eversion occurs superficially, with inferior displacement of the umbilicus and abnormal external genitalia [32]. In classical bladder exstrophy, most of the defects are related to the abdominal wall, pelvic bone, bladder, male genitalia, rectum, and anal canal.

1.4.2.2 Sexuality and fertility concerns for the affected male

Penile length and appearance are the most frequently expressed male concerns in this patient population [33]. Penile lengthening can be achieved with the surgical release of the penile suspensory ligament. If penile skin is not adequate for full coverage of the reconstruction, a full-thickness skin graft can be utilized to substitute the defect [21]. Erectile dysfunction and abnormal ejaculation are commonly encountered in BEEC patients, with the former occurring in up to 63% of patients and the latter affecting up to 41% of patients [31]. The most common causes of sexual dissatisfaction are a short penis, penetration difficulty, and an esthetically displeasing penis [34].

Fertility preservation is not a primary focus during the initial stages of repair in bladder exstrophy [21]. Reynaud et al. investigated the sexuality and fertility of men born with

BEEC. Normal semen parameters were noticed in 7.1% of patients, while 42.9% of patients had azoospermia, and 50% showed other semen parameter abnormalities. Successful pregnancy rates reached 31.6%, with 15.8% of those achieved spontaneously [34].

1.4.3 Prune-belly syndrome

Prune-Belly syndrome (PBS) is a congenital disease defined by the clinical triad of (1) abdominal muscle deficiency, (2) bilateral undescended testes, and (3) urinary tract anomalies. Although the etiology of this disorder is still unknown, multiple theories have been proposed to explain the embryological origin of the disease. The incidence is 3.8 in every 100,000, with a male predominance of around 95% [35]. Clinically, urinary tract anomalies can vary among patients. Though the multiple renal and ureteric anomalies associated with PBS are beyond the scope of this chapter, we will discuss the bladder, prostatic, and testicular anomalies associated with PBS and their impact on the quality of life and fertility potential of male PBS patients.

In PBS patients, the bladder typically appears dilated and hypotonic on voiding cystourethrograms, with the incidence of vesico-uretral reflux reaching 75% of cases. While the bladder is compliant in the urinary storage phase, the hypotonicity leads to incomplete emptying during the voiding phase, which becomes an indication for the diversion of urine [36]. Additionally, the posterior urethra appears dilated due to prostatic hypoplasia [37].

Bilateral undescended testes are classical findings in PBS patients. A recent scoping review also showed that spermatogonia were absent in 50% of testicular histology in PBS patients, while 47.2% had reduced spermatogenesis and only 2.7% had normal sperm production [13]. The review also identified Leydig cell hyperplasia and Sertoli cell-only patterns in 19.4% of male PBS cases. Testosterone levels were normal in 93.9% of patients, while Luteinizing hormone and Follicle-stimulating hormone levels were normal in 87.7 and 77.9% of patients, respectively.

Prostatic hypoplasia and prostatic urethral dilation were also found in 93.6 and 91.4% of patients, respectively, which are thought to be primary contributors to infertility in these patients due to retrograde ejaculation. It was also found that 75.7% of patients had azoospermia and 21.6% were oligospermic. Successful sperm extraction was reported in six cases and resulted in four pregnancies [13]. The data suggest an increased need for fertility assessment, including hormonal profiling and semen analysis in this patient population, with ART increasing the chances of successful pregnancies [13].

In another comparative study of testicular structure in males with PBS, six tissue specimens from the testes of three PBS fetuses and 14 specimens from the testes of non-PBS fetuses were compared and showed no differences in seminiferous tubule numbers and size; however, it was found that PBS testes exhibited a lower number of Leydig cells when compared to the control group, a finding suspected to contribute to the lower sperm production in the male PBS patients [38].

Structural Wolffian duct anomalies are also seen in PBS patients: Absent seminal vesicles and vas deferens, as well as epididymal anomalies. Successful sperm extraction and intracytoplasmic sperm injection can overcome the severe male-factor infertility causes encountered with PBS patients [39].

1.4.3.1 Management

In bladder agenesis patients, the primary goal of treatment is to manage renal impairment, genital reconstruction, and achieve continence. In the early stages of management, patients may need urinary diversion, dialysis, or renal transplantation. Fertility preservation is not an early goal of management. The available literature does not focus on the fertility potential of this population. However, the structural abnormalities in the lower urinary tract are the apparent issues that might affect fertility and sexual life. Spermatogenesis was not documented in any of the previously published cases. Penile reconstruction can help to achieve antegrade ejaculation [40].

Nowadays, patients with bladder exstrophy survive adulthood and raise the desire to father a child; therefore, careful reconstruction must be undertaken to achieve a normal tract with an adequate antegrade ejaculation [41]. Traditionally, BEEC surgical management is approached in a stepwise manner, with the first operation focusing on bladder closure with or without osteotomy. The second operation focuses on urethral reconstruction and epispadias repair. Later, bladder neck reconstruction and ureteral reimplantation are performed to achieve continence. Other approaches described in the literature include two-stage repairs and even a single-stage repair, such as complete primary repair of bladder exstrophy, which intends to reduce the number of operations by closing the bladder and abdominal wall, and bladder neck and epispadias repair, and penile reconstruction in one stage [42].

Berrettini et al. recently published a systematic review on the utilization of substitution phalloplasty, a procedure that utilizes a musculocutaneous flap to reconstruct the penis in BEEC male patients and in other disorders. Their review concentrated on the different techniques in the literature, as well as complications and outcomes. They provide successful reports of augmenting these phalloplasties with penile prostheses to achieve a sexually functional reconstructed phallus, with around 68% of patients in their review receiving this combination to satisfactory outcomes, not just sexually but also esthetically and psychologically. However, the rates of complications in inserting a penile prosthesis in a substitution phallus are higher (up to 25%), including erosion of the prosthesis in 6 of the 47 reviewed patients [43].

Regardless, the notion of substitution phalloplasty, as well as augmenting it with penile prostheses to attain a functional and cosmetic solution in cases of BEEC and PBS, is a leap in the management of the condition. Haddad and her team highlight the importance of such innovative solutions to "ensure BEEC patients and families thrive," including the necessity of multidisciplinary approaches that incorporate medical, surgical, and psychosocial services [44].

1.5 Specific anomalies of the genitalia and the genital tract

1.5.1 Anomalies of the urethra and the penis

Hypospadias is a common congenital anomaly of the penis occurring in approximately 1 in 250 male births. It results from the incomplete fusion of the urethral folds during embryogenesis [45]. This leads to an ectopic urethral meatus on the ventral penis, with the meatal opening occurring anywhere from near the glans to the perineum. Abnormal meatal locations can cause a deflected urinary stream, which could be mild in distal cases, and rarely impair voiding. In contrast, severe proximal cases can cause a downward-directed urinary stream and difficulty in standing to void [46].

Patients with hypospadias also often suffer from a ventral penile curvature, known as chordee, which happens due to fibrous tethering of the penis [46]. Ventral curvature, especially if uncorrected, may lead to painful erections and challenges during sexual intercourse. Men with significant uncorrected curvature or perineal meatus may have abnormal semen deposition, leading to compromised fertility, difficulty achieving intravaginal ejaculation, and in some cases, inability to penetrate [47].

Hypospadias is part of "testicular dysgenesis syndrome," which often occurs with cryptorchidism and low semen quality in some patients [46]. Cryptorchidism occurs in 8–10% of cases [47]. Notably, hypospadias itself does not inherently impair spermatogenesis, and any fertility impact is usually due to mechanical factors or coexisting gonadal anomalies.

Hypospadias is also associated with other genital anomalies, such as inguinal hernias, which occur in about 9–15% of cases [47]. Untreated severe hypospadias can lead to body image concerns and sexual anxiety in adolescence and adulthood, highlighting the importance of the time of surgical correction [48].

Diphallus or penile duplication is an extremely rare congenital anomaly in which a male is born with two penises. It occurs in roughly 1 in 5–6 million live births, with fewer than 120 cases reported [49]. Embryologically, penile duplication results from an abnormal caudal mesenchymal proliferation and cloacal development. Diphallus almost never occurs in isolation; it is usually part of a complex multisystem malformation. Common genitourinary associations include bifid scrotum (split scrotal sac) and urethral duplication (each penis with its own urethra) [49]. There may be duplication of internal structures, such as a double urinary bladder or a duplicated prostate. Cryptorchidism can occur if each hemiphallus has an associated hemiscrotum. Bladder exstrophy and cloacal exstrophy sequence are strongly associated with penile duplication. In such cases, the pubic bones are widely separated, and a diphallus may accompany an exstrophied bladder and intestinal anomalies [49].

1.5.1.1 Management and impact on male reproductive health

The goal of hypospadias repair is to straighten the penis (orthoplasty) and to reconstruct the urethral channel ending at the glans while creating a slit-like, normal-appearing meatus and achieving a good cosmetic outcome (meatoplasty). Surgical correction is typically performed between 6 and 18 months of age for optimal outcomes [50]. Overall, modern hypospadias surgery is highly successful in achieving a straight penis with a terminal meatus. Long-term studies indicate childhood hypospadias repair yields good cosmetic and functional outcomes in adulthood, with normal erectile function scores in the majority of affected men [51].

Management of diphallus is individualized and requires staged reconstructive surgeries [49]. The overarching surgical principle is to retain one functional penis and associated urinary channel while removing or reconstructing the duplicate to ensure one functional genital unit. Typically, the more developed or anatomically correctly positioned phallus is preserved as the primary organ. If one penis has a normal urethral connection to the bladder and the other has an attenuated or no urethra, the latter is usually the one excised.

Phalloplasty is performed to reconstruct and position the remaining penis appropriately on the perineum. Any chordee or penile curvature is corrected during reconstruction. The duplicate penile tissue is excised [49, 52]. The bifid scrotum is repaired by uniting the halves (scrotoplasty) to form a single scrotal pouch. If each penis had an attached testis and hemiscrotum, the testes would be brought together into the reconstructed scrotum. Urethral reconstruction may be needed if the retained penis has an abnormal meatus (e.g., hypospadias repair on the remaining penis). Staged surgeries are common, and the end goal is a single penis capable of normal urination in the standing position and eventual sexual function, with as normal an appearance as possible.

The important notion is that a majority of hypospadias cases will require some form of surgical intervention, be it early or later, and the outcomes of these procedures can affect urinary and sexual function [53]. In isolated hypospadias, testicular function (spermatogenesis and hormonal production) is typically normal, so fertility issues are usually due to anatomical factors. Early surgical repair is a form of fertility preservation: By creating a normally positioned meatus and straightening the penis in infancy, normal erectile function and ejaculation can occur, enabling natural fertility. Men who have had hypospadias repairs should be counseled that overall paternity rates are high and comparable to peers if the repair is successful. However, those with a history of proximal hypospadias, especially if multiple surgeries were needed, may have a slightly higher incidence of sexual dysfunction or ejaculatory disorders in adulthood [54]. It is prudent to follow such patients into adolescence and adulthood (transitional care) to address any erectile curvature recurrence, urethral strictures, or psychological concerns that could affect sexual function.

If a hypospadias patient does experience fertility problems, the approach depends on the cause: Residual curvature can be surgically corrected even in adulthood, and any urethral stricture can be treated to improve ejaculation. ARTs are seldom required solely for hypospadias, but in rare cases of severe, uncorrectable anatomical issues, intrauterine insemination or in vitro fertilization (IVF) can bypass mechanical difficulties. Additionally, in hypospadias associated with dysgenetic testes, early evaluation of fertility potential is recommended [45].

In diphallus, fertility potential depends on the integrity of the testes, vasa deferentia, and the reconstructed genital anatomy [49]. Importantly, most reported diphallus cases have a normal 46, XY karyotype and at least two testicles, often one testis per hemiphallus, or two in a bifid scrotum [49]. If the testes are normally descended or brought into the scrotum during reconstruction and spermatogenesis is normal, there is potential for normal fertility [49]. Surgical management aims to preserve both testes and ensure that at least one functional ejaculatory pathway exists [49]. There is scant literature on long-term fertility outcomes in diphallus due to its rarity [49]. However, if surgical reconstruction results in a single straight penis with a patent urethra, and both testes are present in the scrotum, many patients should be able to ejaculate normally and father children [49].

Fertility preservation in childhood per se (e.g, banking sperm) is not applicable, since patients are prepubertal; instead, the focus is on optimal reconstruction and hormonal monitoring at puberty. As these patients reach adolescence, an assessment of testicular function is necessary. This can include monitoring pubertal development, testicular volume, hormone levels, and, later, semen analysis. In cases where normal intercourse is anatomically feasible but fertility is not achieved, ARTs can be employed [55, 56]. Psychosexual support is also important: Patients with unique genital histories may have anxiety that can affect sexual function, so counseling can improve confidence and thereby indirectly benefit fertility by improving the likelihood of attempted intercourse [56].

1.5.2 Anomalies of the vas deferens and ejaculatory duct

Infertility affects 15% of couples at reproductive age. Male factors are responsible for 50% of the cases. Specifically, azoospermia, which contributes to 15% of male factors, is classified into obstructive and nonobstructive. In obstructive azoospermia, hormones and spermatogenesis are normal, and obstruction is distal to the rete testis [57]. Ejaculatory duct obstruction is uncommon, and it is classified into acquired and congenital. Examples of acquired ejaculatory duct obstruction are seminal vesicle calculi, post-inflammation at the prostate, and a history of urethral trauma. Wolffian duct cysts, Müllerian duct cysts, and ejaculatory duct atresia or stenosis are examples of congenital ejaculatory duct obstruction [58]. The other cause of obstructive azoospermia is a defect in the Wolffian duct, which causes congenital absence of the vas deferens, which is classified into unilateral and bilateral [59].

1.5.2.1 Zinner syndrome

Patients with Zinner syndrome typically present between the ages of 20 and 40 years. The presentation is mostly associated with abdominal pain, obstructive lower urinary tract symptoms, recurrent epididymitis, and infertility due to a large seminal vesicle cyst [60–62]. The initial diagnosis begins with ultrasonography of the kidneys, ureters, and bladder (KUB), which reveals unilateral kidney agenesis and a retrovesical cyst. Transrectal ultrasound offers more detailed information, and magnetic resonance imaging (MRI) is confirmatory [63].

1.5.2.2 Congenital absence of vas deferens

Congenital absence of vas deferens is subdivided into unilateral or bilateral. Congenital unilateral absence of vas deferens (CUAVD) accounts for 0.4% of infertility case; however, congenital bilateral absence of vas deferens (CBAVD) accounts for 1–2%. The most common associated genes with these conditions are cystic fibrosis transmembrane conductance regulator gene (CFTR) and the adhesion G protein-coupled receptor G2 gene (ADGRG2). Up to 46% of CUAVD patients have at least one variant of the CFTR gene [64]. While many patients with this condition can be fertile, some can present with infertility. On the other hand, patients with CBAVD usually present with obstructive azoospermia. Both conditions are associated with upper tract anomalies and are more common with CUAVD. The diagnosis is usually made by physical examination, transrectal ultrasound, and semen analysis. In CUAVD, Semen analysis reveals obstructive azoospermia, oligospermia, or normospermia. In CBAVD, the semen analysis usually shows azoospermia, low pH <7, and low ejaculatory volume [64].

1.5.2.3 Management

Management of seminal vesicle cyst includes transrectal ultrasound-guided aspiration or transurethral resection of the ejaculatory duct obstructing cyst. In large cysts, laparoscopic or robotic surgical cyst excision might be a better option. Studies suggest that surgical intervention improves semen parameters in 63–83% of patients, although persistent azoospermia remains a possibility [63].

In case of CUAVD, the treatment depends on the patency of the contralateral distal vas deferens and the presence of sperm fragments in epididymal fluid. Microsurgical intervention, like vasoepididymostomy, can be used, but these have limited surgical outcomes because of the presence of other anomalies like seminal vesicle agenesis, as these patients have normal spermatogenesis [64]. Assisted reproductive treatment options for persistent azoospermia, seminal vesicle agenesis, and CBAVD include microsurgical epididymal sperm aspiration (MESA), percutaneous epididymal sperm aspiration (PESA), or testicular sperm extraction (TESA) followed by intracytoplasmic injection (ICSI). MESA offers the highest pregnancy rates but carries a risk of transmitting genetic mutations to offspring [65].

The treatment options for ejaculatory duct obstruction include transurethral resection of the ejaculatory duct (TURED), which is the gold standard treatment for ejaculatory duct obstruction and improves semen quality by 59% with a natural pregnancy rate of 12–31%. Complications of this procedure include bladder neck injury and scarring at the ejaculatory duct orifice, leading to persistent azoospermia and epididymorchitis [25].

The other surgical treatment option is transurethral seminal vesiculoscopy, a procedure in which a scope is introduced into the ejaculatory duct to incise or puncture the ejaculatory duct wall. Seminal vesicle obstruction by stones or clots is the main indication for transurethral seminal vesiculoscopy. Seminal vesicle perforation, urethrorectal fistula, and epididymitis are possible complications of this approach, yet these do not overshadow its effectiveness, with one study showing an impressive improvement in semen analysis by 90% [66]. The risk of late obstruction remains a complication in previous approaches. Therefore, ART plays a role in such cases since patients usually have normal spermatogenesis. Thus, PESA, MESA, TESA, and micro-TESA are used to extract the sperm to be used in ICSI, achieving a pregnancy rate of 35% [66].

1.5.3 Undescended testes (cryptorchidism)

Testicular descent from the abdomen is a two-phase process: Transabdominal phase that occurs around 15 weeks of gestation in which the testis migrates to the internal inguinal ring and a subsequent inguinoscrotal phase that is completed by 35 weeks of gestation, where the testis descends through the inguinal canal into the scrotum under the control of testosterone and the genitofemoral nerve release of calcitonin gene-related peptide [46]. Disruption in any of these hormonal or mechanical factors can result in an undescended testis, also known as cryptorchidism.

Cryptorchidism may be unilateral or bilateral, and the testis can be located anywhere along the path of descent or in an ectopic location. Common sites are intra-abdominal, in the inguinal canal, or just above the scrotum; ectopic locations are rare and include the perineal or femoral areas. In many full-term infants with cryptorchidism, the cause is idiopathic. Known risk factors include prematurity, low birth weight, and exposure to environmental estrogenic compounds in utero [46, 67]. Up to 30% of premature boys have at least one undescended testis at birth, but many will descend spontaneously in the first few months of life. By the age of 6 months, the prevalence of cryptorchidism in full-term infants falls to about 1% (from ~3% at birth) due to postnatal descent in some cases [68, 69].

Pathologically, cryptorchid testes show impaired germ cell maturation as early as 6–12 months of age: The normal progression of neonatal gonocytes into adult dark spermatogonia is arrested in undescended testes [70]. Histologically, undescended testes develop fewer total germ cells and Leydig cell abnormalities over time, especially if intra-abdominal, where the warmer temperature causes stress to the seminiferous epithelium. Unilateral cryptorchidism can also adversely affect the contralateral or normally descended testis, possibly *via* shared genetic factors or low-level hormonal aberrations such that even the normal testis may have suboptimal fertility potential [70].

1.5.3.1 Timing and type of intervention-hormonal therapy versus surgical orchiopexy

The cornerstone of cryptorchidism management is early orchiopexy or the surgical placement of the testis into the scrotum. Current guidelines recommend orchiopexy ideally by 18 months of age, and certainly before 2 years of age, to optimize testicular development and future fertility potential [71, 72]. Evidence shows that surgery before 1 year of age results in better germ cell counts and a higher likelihood of normal fertility than surgery after 2–3 years [72–74]. Hormonal therapy for cryptorchidism using human chorionic gonadotrophin (hCG) injections or gonadotrophin-releasing hormone (GnRH) analogs has historically been attempted to induce the testis to descend. hCG mimics luteinizing hormone (LH), thus stimulating Leydig cells to produce testosterone. About 15–20% of undescended testes will transiently descend with hormonal treatment, but many of them may re-ascend. Given the limited efficacy and potential side effects like premature virilization, hormone therapy is not routinely recommended for cryptorchidism by most modern guidelines [74]. An exception is in the context of specific endocrine deficiencies where hormonal therapy is part of treatment, or as an adjunct after orchiopexy in research settings to improve germ cell maturation. Thus, surgery is the definitive therapy for cryptorchidism. Early intervention not only potentially preserves fertility but also may reduce the risk of malignancy (though this risk is not eliminated by orchidopexy) [67]. Notably, if a testis is found to be intra-abdominal, orchiectomy should be considered [75].

1.5.3.2 Impact on fertility

Cryptorchidism is a strong predictor of subfertility in males [73]. Even after orchiopexy, men with a history of undescended testes have, on average, lower sperm counts and reduced fertility compared to men without this history. The degree of impact depends on whether or not cryptorchidism was unilateral or bilateral, and the timing of surgical fixation.

In unilateral cryptorchidism, the majority of men will be fertile, but fertility is still measurably reduced compared to controls [76]. One large study found that among formerly unilateral cryptorchid men who attempted paternity, around 89% were successful compared to 94% of men without cryptorchidism [77]. In contrast, bilateral cryptorchidism has a substantial impact: Paternity rates are around 50–62% even after bilateral orchiopexy, compared to 90% in men without cryptorchidism [76]. In other words, infertility is about six times more frequent in men with bilateral cryptorchidism than in the general population [76]. Notably, if bilateral cryptorchidism is left untreated, nearly all such men will be infertile, with infertility rates exceeding 90% for uncorrected bilateral cases [71].

Unilateral cryptorchidism, if untreated, also carries risk to the fertility of both testes; approximately 10–30% of men with a history of an undescended testis may experience infertility, roughly twice the rate in the general male population [71]. Early orchiopexy improves these odds. Surgery before 1 or 2 years of age can help preserve the testicular germ cell population [70]. However, even with early surgery, some damage may have occurred in utero or in infancy. A key concept is that cryptorchidism can cause bilateral testicular damage even when it occurs unilaterally: The contralateral descended testis often has suboptimal spermatogenesis, and 70% of normal scrotal testes in unilateral cases show impaired maturation of spermatogonia [70, 77]. This suggests a developmental anomaly affecting both testes, perhaps genetically or hormonally mediated. Furthermore, cryptorchidism can be part of the testicular dysgenesis syndrome: A fetal developmental disturbance leading to a spectrum of issues: Undescended testis, hypospadias, poor sperm quality, and increased testicular cancer risk [67].

1.5.3.3 Hormonal function

Most prepubertal boys with unilateral cryptorchidism have normal Leydig cell function and normal testosterone levels at puberty. Bilateral cryptorchidism, though, if uncorrected, can sometimes lead to lower testosterone in adulthood due to diffuse testicular damage, but with timely surgery, many will have normal endocrine function. Serum inhibin B, a marker of Sertoli cell function in childhood, is often reduced in cryptorchid boys, especially if bilateral, predicting lower sperm count later in life [70].

1.5.3.4 Fertility preservation and options

The primary strategy to preserve fertility in cryptorchidism is early bilateral orchiopexy. By placing the testes in the cooler scrotal environment during infancy, further degeneration of germ cells is mitigated [70]. Orchiopexy before 18 months is associated with higher germ cell counts at biopsy and a better chance of spermatogenesis in adulthood compared to late orchiopexy [70]. For patients who had orchiopexy later in childhood or who had high intra-abdominal testes, proactive fertility counseling is important. Once the patient reaches adolescence, an assessment of fertility potential can be made: Testicular volume, hormonal assays, and, eventually, a semen analysis in late teenage years may be necessary. If semen abnormalities are detected, early referral to a reproductive urologist or fertility specialist is warranted.

Men with a history of cryptorchidism and infertility can still achieve biological fatherhood with ART. Intracytoplasmic sperm injection (ICSI) has revolutionized treatment for male-factor infertility; even men with very low sperm counts (oligospermia) or nonobstructive azoospermia can often father children with ICSI if sperm can be retrieved. In men with azoospermia post-cryptorchidism, surgical sperm retrieval from the testes (testicular sperm extraction, TESE, or micro-TESE) can find sperm in a significant proportion of cases. A meta-analysis found that men with nonobstructive azoospermia due to cryptorchidism had higher sperm retrieval success rates when compared to those with idiopathic nonobstructive azoospermia, indicating that focal areas of spermatogenesis often exist in cryptorchid testes [78, 79]. Thus, even if a semen analysis shows no sperm, these patients should be offered TESE rather than assuming absolute infertility.

For adolescents with bilateral cryptorchidism or anyone at high risk of azoospermia, sperm banking in early adulthood, if any ejaculated sperm are present, could be discussed as a precaution [78, 79]. In the future, there is hope for fertility preservation, even earlier experimental protocols aiming to cryopreserve testicular tissue in childhood (containing spermatogonial stem cells) for later re-transplantation or *in vitro* maturation, although this remains investigational [80].

Hormonal therapy in adolescence, such as gonadotropins, guidelines did not mention long-term fertility outcomes [81]. Besides fertility, an important aspect of long-term care is cancer surveillance: Cryptorchidism increases the risk of testicular germ cell tumor fourfold [82]. Orchiopexy somewhat reduces this risk but does not normalize it, especially if done after puberty [82]. Therefore, men with a history of undescended testes should be educated on testicular self-examination and possibly have regular follow-ups [69]. From a fertility standpoint, if one testis is severely damaged or removed, the remaining testis can often maintain normal testosterone and sometimes adequate sperm for natural fertility, but if fertility is impaired, options include ART [55].

2. Neuro-urological conditions and male reproductive health

Neuro-urological conditions are a status that should be explored separately from the resultant neurogenic genito- and lower urinary tract dysfunction that occurs with some, if not a significant proportion, of urological congenital malformations of the lower urinary tract, particularly those of the bladder. These patients represent a special population: Ones who were previously normal in sexual and ejaculatory function, but as a result of a neurological condition such as multiple sclerosis, cerebrovascular accidents, or trauma, experienced newfound dysfunction, often extending beyond neurological erectile dysfunction and involving hormonal and psychogenic changes and effects.

2.1 Multiple sclerosis

2.1.1 Pathophysiology

Multiple sclerosis (MS) is an autoimmune disorder caused by autoreactive immune cells that traverse the blood-brain barrier and attack the central nervous system. This leads to the formation of plaques in the central nervous system together with demyelination, inflammation, axonal loss, and axonal damage. According to Dighriri et al., the plaques are found in the brain and spinal cord, particularly in the white matter around the ventricles, corpus callosum, optic nerves and tracts, and cerebral peduncles. With MS, the consistent deletion of autoreactive immune cells takes place in the thymus or bone marrow through the central tolerance of B cells [83].

2.1.2 Impact on male fertility

MS is common in younger males when they are at their optimal point in life and are ready to start families and have children. According to Geng et al. [84], young males between the ages of 20 and 40 are vulnerable to MS. Men with MS are more likely to experience sexual and reproductive problems [84]. Based on a review of 34 studies, common issues among males with MS are erectile dysfunction, sexual dysfunction, and infertility [85]. Geng et al. [84] support this by revealing that when physicians are handling cases of males with MS, they often encounter sexual and reproductive problems, mainly erectile dysfunction, ejaculatory disorders, decreased sperm quality, lower libido, and impaired fertility. This is mainly because MS causes neurological disability, including sensory dysfunction, fatigue, spasticity, and cognitive dysfunction. Additionally, chronic inflammation, autoimmunity, the use of drugs such as antiepileptic drugs, and psychological factors in males with MS can lead to infertility [85].

In MS, lower urinary tract symptoms (LUTS) and sexual dysfunction progress with disease burden. A study by Redelman showed that 74% of male MS patients had sexual dysfunction, with erectile dysfunction and decreased libido being the most common, and only 29% had access to medical care to help with these difficulties [86]. Multidisciplinary care involving neurologists, urologists, and psychologists led to significantly improved quality of life and better sexual satisfaction scores. Antimuscarinics, mirabegron, and botulinum toxin injections were effective in bladder management, while PDE5 inhibitors improved erectile function in over 60% of treated men. Several centers now advocate for fertility counseling early in the MS trajectory, particularly prior to initiating immunomodulatory therapies known to affect spermatogenesis [87, 88].

2.2 Fertility factors

MS affects sexual and reproductive function in males. Factors implicated include hypogonadotropic hypogonadism, which occurs due to damage to the central nervous system and changes to the hypothalamus-pituitary gland functions. Alternatively, MS patients may suffer from hypergonadotropic hypogonadism, which is a result of low levels of testosterone and reduction of its protective role, as well as autoimmunity. Hypogonadism is common in men with MS, lowering fertility. Additionally, chronic inflammation of the central nervous system leads to semen alterations, and demyelination causes sexual dysfunction [89]. MS patients also experience reduced sexual desire, motivation, excitement, and pleasure. Since MS primarily impacts young people, sexual dysfunction is also another common concern in this population. Patients experience reduced sexual desire and motivation. Additionally, men with MS experience low feelings of sexual arousal and pleasure [90, 91]. The treatment of sexual dysfunction needs multidisciplinary teamwork and cooperation among specialists, working with the individual patients, and raising societal awareness overall [91].

2.3 Spinal cord injury

2.3.1 Pathophysiology

A spinal cord injury (SCI) is a disabling condition that disrupts sensory, motor, and autonomic nervous processes. SCI is reported to affect almost 1 million people every year. SCI damage can be divided into traumatic and nontraumatic. The latter takes place when an acute or chronic condition, such as an infection, tumor, or degenerative disease, causes damage to the spinal cord. Traumatic SCI, as the name suggests, results from a traumatic impact that dislocates or fractures the vertebrae. The most common form of primary impact SCI is compressional vertebral bone injury [92].

2.3.2 Impact on fertility

Young men are the most likely to experience SCI, with young males aged between 16 and 30 years of age being four times more likely to sustain SCI compared to females. SCI affects male fertility through disruptions in the patient's erectile, endocrine, and sexual functions. It leads to poor spermatogenesis and abnormal ejaculation in males as well as erectile dysfunction. Among SCI patients, the most consistent finding on semen analysis is decreased mobility and vitality [93].

Male patients with SCI often face dual challenges of erectile dysfunction and anejaculation. A prospective study on men with SCI conducted by the Miami Project to Cure Paralysis found that penile vibratory stimulation (PVS) achieved ejaculation in 86% of patients with injuries above T10. Sperm retrieval *via* this method resulted in appropriate motile sperm counts suitable for intrauterine insemination (IUI) in 71% of ejaculates. Importantly, fertility counseling and andrology referral improved utilization of these options [94]. Furthermore, a 10-year follow-up from a Florence-based rehabilitation program showed that early penile rehabilitation with the use of PDE5 inhibitors correlated with better long-term satisfaction and improved partner intimacy among injured men [95].

Reports discuss several theories for the abnormal sperm mobility, including high scrotal temperature, antisperm antibodies, leukospermia, and seminal plasma proteins and cytokines. Findings of ejaculate discoloration after SCI have also been reported, though correlation to impaired fertility function is not established. There are also recent reports that there are different inflammatory protein complexes activated in SCI patients that affect semen parameters. These so-called "inflammasomes" may be a potential treatment target in the future [96].

Beyond altered semen analysis parameters, SCI also causes infertility by causing neurogenic and psychogenic forms of erectile dysfunction. Normally, erections in males are either psychogenic or reflex. Both forms of erection rely on the lower motor sacral nerves being intact. When SCI occurs and there is complete injury above T11, the patient may not be able to develop or sustain erections. Due to SCI, the highly coordinated processes of erection, emission, and ejaculation can be disrupted at any step, and without any medical intervention, can result in sexual dysfunction and infertility [93, 97].

2.3.3 Factors to consider

Based on the impact of SCI on male fertility, it is apparent that SCI affects almost every aspect of the male reproductive process. SCI also leads to decreased sperm motility regardless of the patient having a normal sperm count, as well as abnormal semen ejaculation and emission. Therefore, when developing treatment strategies for men with SCI, we must target these various dysfunctions (**Table 1**).

2.4 Cerebrovascular accident

2.4.1 Pathophysiology

A cerebrovascular accident (CVA) or a "stroke" is a medical state attributed to acute compromise of the cerebral perfusion or vasculature. The primary cause of strokes is hypertension; however, in young adults, carotid dissection, clotting disorders, and substance abuse are other common causes [98].

2.4.2 Impact on fertility

Stroke is considered a global health issue, with high mortality and disability rates [99]. Men of reproductive age and potential who experience a stroke generally are affected by hyposexuality, which is a decline in desire for sexual activity. After a stroke, a patient can face challenges of insecurity and recovery, which lowers their desire for sex. Medications such as antidepressants can also decrease the individual's sex drive. Following a stroke, libido usually decreases, and the prevalence of low sexual desire is reported to be between 17 and 42%. Additionally, erectile dysfunction is higher in males who have suffered a stroke [100, 101]. Nevertheless, this association was related to the age of the patient and the age at which the CVA may have occurred, rather than associations with other classically causative and modifiable cardiovascular risk factors of erectile dysfunction [102].

Post-stroke patients frequently report urinary urgency, incontinence, and reduced libido. A cohort study by Montalvan et al. involving 150 men post-CVA showed that 59% had new-onset sexual dysfunction within months of surviving. Erectile dysfunction was significantly associated with total infarctions of the anterior circulation and

Congenital anomaly	Impact on fertility	Management options	Role of ART
CAKUT (e.g., renal agenesis, ureteral duplication)	Hypogonadism, abnormal seminal vesicles, ejaculatory duct obstruction	Urological reconstruction, endocrine management	Case dependent
Bladder exstrophy	Ejaculatory dysfunction, shortened penis, abnormal semen parameters	Surgical reconstruction (bladder neck, epispadias repair), hormonal support	Often needed, e.g., ICSI
Prune belly syndrome	Cryptorchidism, azoospermia, hypoplastic vas deferens	Orchiopexy, hormonal therapy, sperm retrieval (micro-TESE)	Frequently required
Posterior urethral valves	Secondary damage to testes, possible retrograde ejaculation	Valve ablation, long-term renal and testicular monitoring	Sometimes needed depending on ejaculatory function
Hypospadias	Indirect, mostly erectile dysfunction if not repaired	Reconstruction	Case dependent
Cryptorchidism	Variable, impaired sometimes despite orchidopexy	Orchidopexy, orchidectomy	May be needed
Spina Bifida/ Myelomeningocele	Anejaculation, erectile dysfunction, low sperm count	Penile prosthesis, vibroejaculation or electroejaculation, sperm retrieval	Commonly required for biological fertility

Table 1.
Summary of male congenital genito-urinary anomalies and fertility management.

previous CVAs [103]. While spontaneous could occur in some cases, the introduction of PDE5 inhibitors, pelvic floor physiotherapy, and psychosexual support programs led to improved outcomes [101]. Importantly, stroke rehabilitation clinics that included sexual health screening and urology referral reported higher patient satisfaction and improved partner dynamics, especially in younger men seeking fertility after stroke recovery [100, 104].

2.5 Management

Erectile dysfunction, reduced libido, ejaculatory dysfunction, and fatigue are the common issues for males with MS (**Figure 2**). In 2021, a European case study revealed that 70% of men with MS reported anejaculation and 50% had abnormal sperm parameters [87]. One of the main barriers is the need to manage these conditions through multisystem involvement. Managing MS needs the integration of neurology, endocrinology, urology, and psychology. Getting to coordinate each of these units is a challenge in the management of MS. In addition, there is the psychological impact, which will be discussed somewhere else in the chapter. Management of sexual dysfunction among males with MS starts with a comprehensive assessment, including neurological evaluation, sexual history, and the use of tools such as the International Index of Erectile Function (IIEF-5). In instances of anejaculation or retrograde ejaculation, penile vibratory stimulation (PVS) and electroejaculation (EEJ) are noninvasive and effective methods for sperm retrieval, mainly in those aiming to attain fertility [105].

Hormonal evaluation is essential, and testosterone replacement therapy may be beneficial in men with MS-related hypogonadism. Psychosexual therapy, including

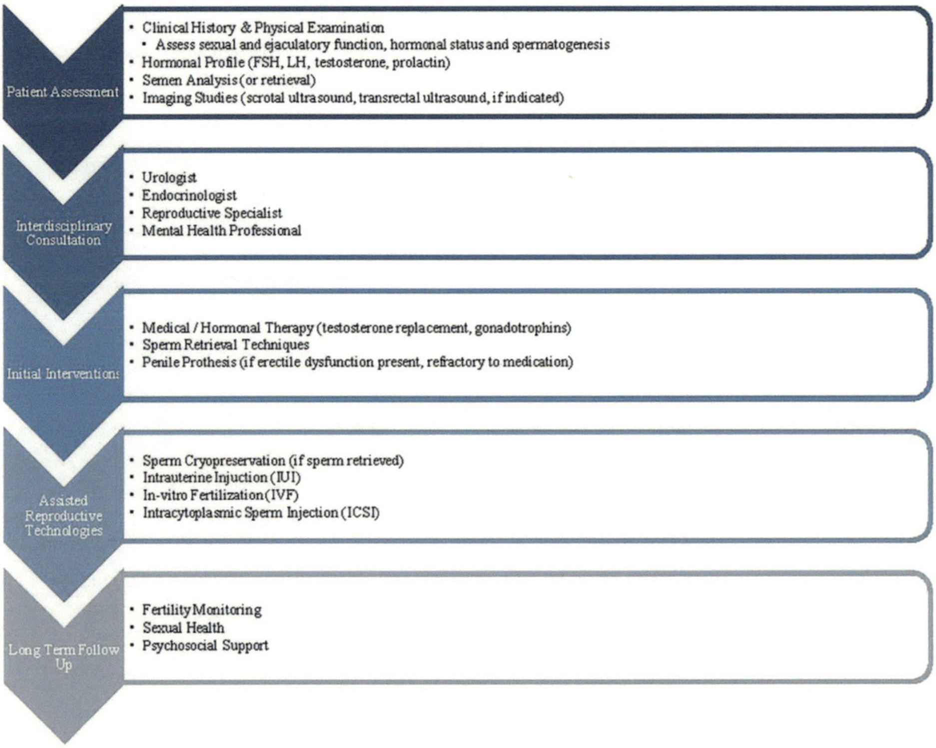

Figure 2.
Suggested flowchart of workup of neurological patients with reproductive issues.

cognitive-behavioral therapy and relationship counseling, plays a valuable role in addressing tertiary sexual dysfunction.

In patients with CVA, managing sexual dysfunction presents various challenges, including the patient's reluctance to discuss the issue, feeling embarrassed, and limited time and knowledge among healthcare professionals. Based on a study of the return of patients who have suffered a stroke to sexual activity, the majority of the males who participated in the study reported initial difficulty going back to normal sexual activities, and two-thirds stated it took 7 weeks to engage in a sexual activity again [7]. The management of sexual dysfunction in males following a stroke needs a multidisciplinary approach. The approach addresses the complex interplay between hormonal, neurological, vascular, and psychological factors. The first step involves thorough assessment through validated tools such as IIEF-5 and hormonal profiling to identify hypogonadism or other endocrine abnormalities [101, 106].

Psychological support is central, as post-stroke depression, anxiety, and altered body image significantly led to sexual difficulties. As a result, cognitive-behavioral therapy (CBT) and couples counseling are recommended as first-line interventions. Next, pharmacological therapy, mainly phosphodiesterase-5 (PDE5) inhibitors such as sildenafil or tadalafil, is considered the center of treatment for erectile dysfunction, provided there are no contraindications such as concurrent nitrate use [107]. For patients unresponsive to medications, non-pharmacological options such as vacuum erection devices, intracorneal injections, or surgical implantation of penile prostheses can be used.

DOI: http://dx.doi.org/10.5772/intechopen.1012843

In the management process of male patients recovering from spinal cord injury, studies reveal that most men felt their injury had affected their sexual sense [105]. However, there are barriers to sexual health. For example, evidence suggests one main issue is the lack of inpatient and community-based sexual rehabilitation centers [108]. Secondly, there is little consensus about how and who ought to address the issues of sexual dysfunction and infertility in men with spinal cord injuries [108]. Therefore, effective management is necessary for males with spinal cord injuries who also face sexual dysfunction issues.

In the management of factors such as erectile dysfunction, PDE5 inhibitors such as sildenafil or tadalafil are effective in men with preserved sacral reflexes. If PDE5 inhibitors are ineffective, vacuum erection devices, intracavernosal injections of prostaglandins, or penile prostheses may be applied [109]. Ejaculatory dysfunction, especially in those with upper motor neuron lesions, can often be managed using PVS. For those who do not respond to PVS, EEJ under anesthesia can be used to retrieve sperm for assisted reproductive techniques. In men looking for fertility, ART, such as intrauterine insemination (IUI), *in vitro* fertilization (IVF), or intracytoplasmic sperm injection (ICSI), are employed depending on semen quality [109].

3. Spinal dysraphism

Spinal dysraphism is a special congenital group of disorders that presents with a distinct set of neurological genitourinary symptoms and conditions. Its pathophysiology, signs and symptoms, and sequelae differ from other urological congenitalisms and neuro-urological conditions, though management principles, particularly with respect to fertility and sexual function, may essentially overlap [110, 111].

3.1 Pathophysiology

Spinal dysraphism refers to a group of diverse conditions that have different imaging patterns. It involves a spectrum of congenital anomalies that cause a defective neural arch through which neural elements are herniated, causing a variety of clinical manifestations [112]. Congenital anomalies are defined as functional or structural abnormalities that take place during the intrauterine life. Spinal dysraphism, it results from aberrations in the closely connected embryological process taking place between gestational weeks two and six, namely, gastrulation (2–3 weeks), primary neurulation (3–4 weeks), and secondary neurulation (5–6 weeks) [113]. In the first 2 months of gestation, the neural plate is formed around the 18th day, which is followed by neural folds and their fusion. By day 28, the expansion of the neural tube and its subsequent closure occur. Open defects take place when the caudal neuropore fails to close. The spinal cord formation is set by the secondary neurulation process. Defects at this phase cause occult dysraphism. The level of coordination between these processes elucidates why the abnormal development of one structure will be linked to the maldevelopment of the other [113].

The clinical manifestations of spinal dysraphism are classified into two: Visible lesions and closed spinal dysraphism (CSD). The latter lacks external lesions. In CSD, the overlying skin is intact; however, the spinal cord is anchored to different tissues beginning from the skin, subcutaneous tissue, and adipose tissue. A combination of genetic and environmental factors causes spinal dysraphism. In the visible lesions, neural tissue is exposed through a defect in the skin and vertebrae. Common types include myelomeningocele, which is a herniation of the spinal cord and meninges, and myelocele, an exposed spinal cord without meninges. The estimated incidence of spinal dysraphism is approximately 1–3/1000 live births [113]. On a positive note, the condition has been on the decline around the world in the past few decades due to improved nutrition among women. Improved antenatal care, folic acid supplementation, and improved ultrasound for prenatal screening are some of the factors contributing to the decline of spinal dysraphism around the globe.

The pathophysiology of spinal dysraphism has various consequences, including neurological dysfunction, hydrocephalus, tethered cord syndrome, and high infection risk. Within the neurological dysfunction is where male infertility comes in. This is because spinal dysraphism can cause weakness or paralysis of the lower limbs and sensory defects.

3.2 Impact on male fertility

Overall, infertility is a result of defects in spermatogenesis or failure of the sperm to move. In connection with spinal dysraphism, few studies have been done to evaluate the impact of spinal dysraphism on male fertility. In one study involving 12 men with spinal dysraphism, the researchers found that only one of the six men who participated in the study was able to successfully become a father [114]. In a different study, 13% out of a sample of 18 men with spinal dysraphism engaged in sexual intercourse, and only one person achieved fatherhood [115]. These data reveal a significant connection between spinal dysraphism and male infertility. While patients have intact libido, men with spinal dysraphism face barriers to fatherhood, including erectile dysfunction, poor sperm quality, anejaculation, and social and/or physical limitations [110].

Spermatogenetic defects are one of the broadly classified causes of infertility. Spermatogenetic defects mostly lead to poor sperm quality and may be linked to a marked decrease in spermatogenetic cells. Based on a study by Hulting et al., semen examined from nine males with spinal dysraphism, aged between 22 and 39, showed that 5 of the 9 men had enough sperm. The other four had extremely low sperm count, and only one of the five men had more than 10,000 live sperm on semen evaluation [116]. The findings of this study, albeit small, reveal that neurological dysfunction declines the production of sperm in men, which creates the link between spinal dysraphism and male infertility.

Aside from spermatogenetic defects, the other class of factors that lead to male infertility the failure of sperm to transport. Within this class is erectile dysfunction. The level of neurological lesion impacts the rate of erectile dysfunction. For example, 36% of men with lesions at or below T10 and 86% of men with lesions above T10 suffer from erectile dysfunction [117]. Men with spinal dysraphism mostly have successful erections and are able to engage in sexual intercourse. However, when asked, only a small number are satisfied with the level of rigidity. This therefore suggests that the majority of perceived erections may be small for intercourse and thus delivery of sperm.

Still, sperm delivery is a form of ejaculatory dysfunction. Many patients with spinal dysraphism suffer from ejaculatory dysfunction, which includes conditions such as retrograde ejaculation and anejaculation. Men with spinal dysraphism do experience ejaculation; however, the delivery is weak and mostly a drip-like emission [114]. Furthermore, about 20% of men with spinal dysraphism lack sensory innervation, hence they fail to perceive ejaculation. Men with tethered cords as a result of spinal dysraphism may experience retrograde ejaculation due to bladder neck incompetence [114].

In a study involving men aged between 13 and 28 suffering from spinal dysraphism, the subjects reported they felt that their physical condition was a hindrance to sexual intercourse. In this case, the physical condition involves being bound to a wheelchair, having to use crutches, and wearing leg braces. Other impediments to sexual intercourse are psychological, including patients feeling they lack self-confidence and being dependent on others, which makes them unable to pursue and maintain romantic relationships. Last, urinary incontinence creates embarrassment, which may contribute to poor social performance and high anxiety when it comes to sexual interactions.

For patients with spinal dysraphism, the main factor to consider is the level of spinal cord lesions, which determines the extent of deficits, fertility, and sexual function [118]. Many studies have linked lower spinal cord lesions with less severe neurological deficits and thus more sexual function. According to research, 64% of men with lesions at T10 or lower had erections, while 14% with lesions above T10 also had erections. Studies show that infertility in men with spinal dysraphism is higher in men with higher lesions. This is possibly attributed to more than just ejaculatory and erectile dysfunction, since these men were also at a high risk of azoospermia [111]. In a study by Reilly and Oates, 10 men with erectile dysfunction had azoospermia following electroejaculation. Their testicular biopsies showed Sertoli cell histology [119].

Another factor to consider is hydrocephalus, which affects more than 85% of infants with spinal dysraphism. Hydrocephalus causes infertility and dysfunction. People with hydrocephalus have fewer relationships, and they have less sexual activity. Men with hydrocephalus reported reduced sexual excitement, ejaculation, orgasm, and erection compared to those without [118].

The fertility options for men with spinal dysraphism include pharmacological and surgical strategies aimed at targeting specific aspects of infertility. In erectile dysfunction, men with spinal dysraphism can use PDE5 inhibitors to improve erections. In a randomized study, men with erectile dysfunction due to spinal dysraphism were administered 20 and 50 mg sildenafil an hour before sex, which led to significant improvements in erectile function [120]. In the same study, researchers revealed that the patients also experienced sexual confidence.

In ejaculatory dysfunction, which is also a significant cause of infertility, urologists use rectal probe electroejaculation under general anesthesia. This method is considered effective for collecting semen, from which viable sperm can be isolated [118]. For men experiencing retrograde ejaculation, the surgical retrieval of sperm from the genitourinary tract, which includes the testicle, epididymis, and vas deferens, is considered more effective in order to collect sperm for ART. The surgical approach for both erectile and ejaculatory dysfunction also aims to enhance penile sensation.

Last, there is the ART approach, which involves the manipulation of embryos to enhance the chances of successful fertilization. There are various methods of ARTs, and they all need some level of baseline spermatogenesis [118]. With the innovation of *in vitro* fertilization, an embryo can be derived from two gametes in a controlled lab. Furthermore, intrauterine insemination, which is also another form of ART, has the probability of enhancing success in fertilization.

4. Contemporary management approaches

Management of these patient populations extends beyond organic treatment of erectile dysfunction or hormonal imbalances and often requires approaches that involve and target a more holistic approach to optimize outcomes of more traditional managements.

4.1 Personalized nutrition as a supportive strategy

Men with congenital urological anomalies, a history of reconstructive surgery, or neuro-urological conditions often face fertility challenges. Creating an adequate nutritional plan may support their reproductive health [121, 122]. Furthermore, affecting hormone levels and spermatogenesis [121]. A personalized nutrition approach to an individual's needs correcting micronutrient deficiencies or metabolic issues that impair fertility [121]. For example, genetic differences in nutrient metabolism (nutrigenetics) may impact sperm quality and DNA-based dietary plans are being explored to enhance male fertility individually [121].

Adherence to a healthy diet pattern, antioxidant diet is associated with improving semen parameters, better metabolic health, reduced oxidative stress and sustaining an optimal body weight [122]. Genetic testing, microbiome analysis, and personalized coaching help doctors to create custom diet and supplement plans [122]. These plans target specific issues, such as oxidative stress or hormonal imbalances that may affect fertility [122]. This personalized strategy complements by creating an optimal environment for spermatogenesis and overall reproductive health [121, 122].

4.2 Lifestyle modifications to enhance fertility and reproductive health

Other lifestyle modifications play role in male fertility. Regular physical activity is highly beneficial. A study shows that resistance exercise significantly improved semen volume, sperm count, motility, and morphology in men [123]. Obesity is linked with low testosterone levels and poor sperm quality [122, 124]. On the other hand, weight loss through diet and exercise can normalize reproductive hormones and improve semen parameters [122, 124]. Healthy diet and regular exercise are both important for good fertility. Consuming a good amount of seafood, fruits, and vegetables while avoiding processed meats, sugary drinks, and fatty diet help to improve sperm quality and increase chance of getting pregnant [124].

Avoiding harmful substances is important as well. Cigarette smoking and heavy alcohol use have a toxic effects on sperm by increasing DNA fragmentation, reducing count and motility [123, 125]. However, studies show that quitting smoking can lead to notable improvements in sperm concentration, count, and motility within months [123].

Men are advised to cease tobacco use and limit their alcohol intake to support fertility [125]. Other factors include stress and sleep; chronic psychological stress and sleep deprivation may disrupt the hormonal regulation of spermatogenesis, there for, stress reduction techniques and good sleep hygiene are recommended for men experiencing infertility [125].

4.3 Preventive strategies beyond nutrition and lifestyle

Limiting environmental and occupational exposures is essential, as excessive heat (e.g., from hot tubs) and toxins like pesticides and heavy metals negatively affect spermatogenesis [123]. When exposure is unavoidable, protective measures and routine sperm quality monitoring should be implemented [123].

Proactive management of comorbid medical conditions such as diabetes or hypertension is vital, as these conditions can impair fertility through hormonal and vascular pathways. Optimizing treatment of these diseases by managing insulin resistance improves sperm count and motility [123, 125]. Additionally, treatment of urogenital infections also helps protect fertility by preventing reproductive tissue damage [123].

Antioxidant supplements, such as vitamins C and E, coenzyme Q10, and carnitine, help reduce oxidative stress and improve sperm health, especially when oxidative stress is confirmed through tests [121]. Patients with serious physical or nerve problems, such as spinal cord injury or blocked ejaculatory ducts, should be referred early for fertility preservation methods, such as sperm collection and freezing. This ensures they have future options for starting a family, including treatments like IVF [123, 125].

4.4 Challenges and considerations in implementation

Personalized nutritional plans and lifestyle modification may pose difficulties. Men with neuro-urological disabilities or chronic illness may find regular exercise or meal preparation difficult and will need modified programs [126]. Limited time, financial constraints, and uncertainty regarding the effectiveness of lifestyle changes are also barriers some patients encounter [126]. Incorrect information about fertility diet and supplements adds further challenge [126]. Misinformation about fertility diets and supplements adds confusion [126]. To overcome these barriers, it requires clear education to explain how lifestyle changes can improve fertility [126]. A combination of professionals is required to offer great care; this includes experts in dietetics, physical therapy, psychology, and reproductive medicine [126]. Of course, personal preference and cultural background will increase a patient's sense of responsibility [126]. Additionally, insurance benefits can greatly assist in implementation and improve patient outcomes.

5. Surgical reconstruction and impacts on male reproductive health fertility

Surgical reconstruction is a cornerstone in the management of congenital and acquired genital anomalies in males, aiming to restore urinary, sexual, and reproductive function. While the technical aspects of phalloplasty and penile prosthesis implantation are well studied, their implications for fertility—both biological and psychosocial—are often underappreciated. Recent advancements in surgical technique, prosthetic technology, and assisted reproductive medicine have allowed for limited but meaningful fertility success in this cohort, particularly when patients are managed in multidisciplinary settings that include reconstructive urologists, andrologists, and fertility counselors.

Phalloplasty, whether performed for congenital absence, traumatic loss, or gender-affirming surgery, typically involves use of radial forearm free flap (RFFF), anterolateral thigh (ALT) flap, or musculocutaneous latissimus dorsi flap. While these neophalluses can support a neourethra and accommodate prosthetic implantation, they lack internal reproductive structures, limiting the potential for natural ejaculation [127, 128]. Despite these limitations, patient-reported outcome measures (PROMs) from tertiary reconstructive centers consistently show high levels of psychosocial benefit, albeit the reports are of small sample size due to the rarity of these conditions [129, 130]. Beyond the esthetic and functional capacity of the neophallus, biological paternity is possible in phalloplasty patients *via* TESE and ICSI.

Penile prosthesis implantation, most commonly the three-piece inflatable type, serves as a definitive solution for erectile dysfunction in patients with congenital anomalies, neurogenic bladder, or post-reconstructive sexual dysfunction. While these implants restore penetrative ability, they do not affect ejaculatory function or correct upstream reproductive tract anomalies. Nevertheless, PROMs consistently indicate high satisfaction rates with respect to sexual activity, self-esteem, and partner intimacy. In a systematic review of 11 studies and 475 men with spinal cord injury, up to 90% of prosthesis recipients reported improved sexual satisfaction, with similar findings reported by their partners [131]. Although fertility rates were not directly assessed, the improved sexual function created a platform for pursuing assisted ejaculation or sperm retrieval methods.

Fertility-focused PROMs, while less frequently reported, suggest that psychological readiness for parenthood increases following reconstructive milestones. In several studies, adolescent males with bladder exstrophy who underwent penile and urethral reconstruction were significantly more likely to inquire about fertility options than those who deferred reconstruction [132, 133]. Qualitative interviews revealed that restoration of body image and functional anatomy promoted discussions about fatherhood, often for the first time [134, 135]. This reinforces the concept that surgical reconstruction may act as a psychosocial gateway to future fertility planning, especially in patients who previously felt excluded from normative reproductive expectations. It is also important to emphasize that, while natural fertility remains rare in this group, multidisciplinary pathways—including cryopreservation, hormonal optimization, electroejaculation, and microsurgical sperm retrieval—can yield meaningful results [136, 137].

In essence, phalloplasty and penile prosthesis implantation significantly enhance sexual function and quality of life, and while they do not directly restore fertility, they facilitate its pursuit through psychosocial and anatomical empowerment. Integrating fertility assessment, patient-reported outcome tracking, and access to ART into surgical planning is essential to ensure that the reconstructive journey addresses not just form and function but also the fundamental human desire for parenthood.

6. Transition urology and the role of multidisciplinary teams in optimizing reproductive and fertility outcomes

As survival rates improve and life expectancy increases among children with congenital urological and neuro-urological conditions, the focus of care must evolve accordingly. These patients are no longer limited to pediatric milestones alone; they grow into adolescence and adulthood with complex, often lifelong anatomical and functional challenges. Transition urology has emerged to meet this need, offering a structured framework that ensures continuity of care across the pediatric-adult divide. More than just a logistical handover, this process entails a shift in care philosophy—from a parent-driven, protective healthcare model to one that is patient-centered, autonomous, and holistic. It also entails tailoring care to reduce complications as survival increases, monitoring for potential malignancies, as well as preparing the adult with urological congenitalism for sexuality and potential fertility (Basics of transition urology). The transition period is therefore a critical window where reproductive and fertility health must be actively reviewed, discussed, and optimized as part of a wider long-term care plan [138–140].

Adolescence is a period when sexuality, identity, and fertility potential begin to carry greater personal and social significance. Yet, for many patients with congenital urological anomalies such as bladder exstrophy, posterior urethral valves, prune belly syndrome, or neurogenic bladder, fertility counseling is often delayed, fragmented, or absent altogether. Formal transition clinics provide a much-needed platform to address these gaps. Structured programs that introduce the concept of fertility preservation early—through hormonal profiling, semen analysis, and timely referrals to reproductive specialists—empower patients with informed choices. For patients with neuro-urological conditions such as multiple sclerosis or spinal cord injuries, transition clinics also serve to coordinate assessments of erectile function, ejaculation, and sperm viability, facilitating early planning for ART when indicated. This anticipatory approach allows for proactive management rather than reactionary care in adulthood [138–141].

Critically, the success of any transition model relies on the presence and functionality of a well-coordinated multidisciplinary team. Pediatric patients are often managed within unified, integrated pediatric centers. In contrast, adult services tend to be more fragmented, requiring collaboration between different departments, institutions, and specialists. Urologists with expertise in functional, reconstructive, and neuro-urology must collaborate with nephrologists, endocrinologists, colorectal surgeons, fertility specialists, psychologists, continence nurses, and social workers. This collaborative model is essential not only for complex surgical planning and bladder function preservation but also for long-term reproductive health. Fertility optimization is no longer a luxury in this cohort—it is a necessary domain of care, particularly in light of emerging evidence on subfertility rates and ejaculatory dysfunction in males with congenital urological anomalies [138–144].

Several structured transition urology models have been reported internationally, with notable success in managing congenital male urological conditions and lifelong neuro-urological disorders. The University of Oklahoma Health Sciences Center model is among the most well-defined, employing a staged approach (T1–T4) beginning in early adolescence. This model gradually introduces patients and their families to adult care processes, with shared consultations between pediatric and adult urologists before formal handover. Their 9-year prospective experience in patients with congenital neurogenic bladder reported a transition success rate of 96%, reinforcing the value of early planning, structured readiness assessments, and continuity in urological oversight [143].

Similarly, a recently published collaborative model between the Royal Children's Hospital and the Royal Melbourne Hospital in Victoria, Australia, exemplifies a regionally adapted yet robust framework. Initiated by age 15, the process includes needs-based multidisciplinary meetings, joint outpatient clinics attended by both pediatric and adult urologists, and collaborative operating for complex cases. Among their cohort of transitioned patients, most of whom had conditions such as spina bifida, posterior urethral valves, and bladder exstrophy, over 90% remained in specialist adult urology care. A substantial proportion required further surgical intervention or renal support, affirming the importance of specialized adult services familiar with congenital and neuro-urological conditions [138]. These models highlight that when transition is coordinated, multidisciplinary, and patient-centered, long-term urological outcomes—including fertility and sexual function—can be preserved and optimized well into adulthood.

Our experience, and that of the aforementioned and other structured programs internationally, confirms that the integration of transition pathways with multidisciplinary involvement leads to improved outcomes. From many transition urology models, transition success rates exceed 90%, yet significant proportions of patients still require many surgical revisions, fertility interventions, or enhanced psychosocial support during the early years of adult follow-up. The ability to maintain a seamless continuum of care during this vulnerable stage of life ensures that patients are not lost to follow-up or left with unresolved issues impacting their reproductive future. In essence, transition and adolescent urology serve not only to uphold the surgical and functional gains of childhood but to facilitate adult autonomy, sexual health, and the potential for biological parenthood—goals that are deeply meaningful to patients and should be central to modern urological care [138, 143–145].

In neuro-urological patients with acquired conditions such as multiple sclerosis, spinal cord injury, and cerebrovascular accidents, multidisciplinary care is equally crucial. These patients often experience overlapping dysfunctions—including erectile dysfunction, ejaculatory disorders, fatigue, spasticity, and mood disturbances—that directly or indirectly impair fertility and sexual well-being. A siloed urological approach is insufficient. Instead, urologists must coordinate care with neurologists for disease-modifying therapies, physiatrists for motor rehabilitation, endocrinologists for testosterone optimization, and mental-health professionals for the management of depression and intimacy-related distress. Fertility specialists must be engaged early to assess reproductive potential and offer options for cryopreservation or assisted reproduction. This integrated model is not just ideal—it is essential to adequately address the multifactorial impact of neuro-urological disease on sexual and reproductive health [84, 85, 89, 90, 93, 99, 100, 138, 146–149].

Moreover, tailored counseling and adaptive interventions should form the cornerstone of long-term follow-up in this population. Men with spinal cord injuries, for example, may require a combination of phosphodiesterase inhibitors, intracavernosal injections, and penile prostheses not only to restore sexual function but also to facilitate independence in catheterization or intercourse. Similarly, post-stroke patients with psychogenic or vascular erectile dysfunction require nuanced care pathways that align with their neurological recovery. The collaborative input of rehabilitation physicians, speech and occupational therapists, and sexuality counselors ensures that treatment plans are not only medically sound but also sensitive to the broader context of the patient's functional status and personal aspirations. Multidisciplinary fertility care is therefore not an adjunct to neuro-urology—it is a vital extension of it [138, 141–143].

7. Ethical and psychosocial dimensions of care

Patients with congenital and neuro-urological disease experience a unique challenge, which extends beyond the anatomical, functional, and sexual dysfunction. The ongoing psychosocial challenge requires a proper identification of the problem and dedicated management once applicable [150–152]. On the other hand, the decision-making in this specific age group is also different whether regarding pediatric patients facing a potentially affected fertility/sexuality or even an adult patient with impaired mental capacity to make a decision.

In this part, we raise the importance of the ethical and psychosocial aspects of this population.

7.1 Ethical considerations in fertility preservation (FP)

FP can be offered for any patient with potentially affected fertility, including spina bifida, Cerebral palsy, Disorders of sex development, Prune Belly syndrome, Hypospadias, Bladder exstrophy-epispadias, and complex spinal cord injuries [153]. Obtaining informed consent for FP in pediatric patients presents a unique challenge; prepubertal boys are not legally or mentally able to provide full informed consent for FP options in which the parents or guardians are the main decision makers at that point. Thus, involving the parents or guardians in the discussion of FP is crucial [154]. This could be challenging due to the unknown desire to preserve fertility in this age group especially in the presence of invasive FP techniques such as testicular tissue cryopreservation in cases of impaired ejaculation [155]. Assessing decision-making capacity is also an important step prior to initiation of this discussion. For example, in the case of traumatic brain injury, that might impair the cognitive abilities of the individual. Therefore, it is crucial to involve the partner or representative in an ongoing discussion about whether FP should be done or not [156]. Timing to initiate FP discussion with the patient or guardians is also crucial. The European association of urology guidelines stated that "Patients and caregivers should be informed not only about the impact of gonadotoxic treatments on future fertility, but also about fertility-preservation options and their risk-benefit ratio. There are also a number of non-oncological congenital anomalies where fertility preservation can become an issue" [157].

When applicable, semen fluid-based cryopreservation by masturbation or penile vibration is the best option. However, in very difficult circumstances, electroejaculation can be discussed. Options like testicular tissue cryopreservation should only be discussed in specific cases by a multidisciplinary team [157].

7.2 Psychosocial impact of infertility and sexual dysfunction

The psychosocial effect of infertility and sexual dysfunction is well recognized. Depression and anxiety are highly related to infertility in both men and women. In a review of 377 related articles, the prevalence of depression, anxiety, and poor QoL is highly relevant to infertility [158]. A systematic review of 309 studies that involved 512 infertile couples concluded that psychiatric intervention improved marital status and sexual satisfaction [159]. Erectile dysfunction plays an important role in the psychosocial status of the patient. A systematic review of 40 articles, which involved 32 randomized controlled trials comparing the psychosocial status of patients treated for erectile dysfunction, showed a great impact of erectile dysfunction and emphasized the importance of treatment on patients' QoL [160].

7.3 Strategies for providing holistic care

The co-existence of sexual dysfunction, infertility, and psychosocial effects of the patient's disease highly affects the patient's QoL, and understanding this critical point gives a higher chance to improve it. Once the psychological diagnosis is made, a multidisciplinary approach will help to decrease the psychological burden on the patient and his/her family, improve fertility potential, and lower the financial burden on the family and the healthcare system by decreasing the investigations or procedures that are not in need. This multidisciplinary approach should include the primary treating physician, urologist, reproductive endocrinologist, social worker, and psychiatrist [159, 161].

8. Future directions and research needs

Nowadays, technologies are well on route to fill the gaps in the management of men with congenital defects and neuro-urological diseases affecting their fertility and their sexual function. Though promising, stem cell therapy, artificial intelligence (AI), and advanced microsurgical techniques are largely experimental and require further research [162].

Studies on animals indicate that stem cell transplant can regenerate sperm-producing tissue and improve fertility parameters; however, there is limited data on outcomes in humans and further studies are needed [163].

In the diagnosis and treatment of infertility, AI has made progress. For instance, AI can analyze huge data in the form of hormonal profiles and sperm micro-imaging to determine possible fertility outcomes [164]. AI self-management software can also improve semen analysis by assisting in leading a healthier lifestyle, while other platforms can provide assistance in making decisions about the diagnosis and treatment of male infertility diseases such as varicoceles [164]. However, these tools require validation to ensure they enhance clinical results without any bias.

Robotic-assisted microsurgery offers benefits due to its accuracy. Robotic systems can eliminate tremor and provide magnified 3D vision for procedures such as vasectomy reversal or varicocelectomy [165]. Studies suggest that these techniques are feasible [165]. However, further trials must confirm whether robot-assisted surgery truly improves success rates or cost-effectiveness over other methods.

In neuro-urology, new treatments are emerging that aim to overcome nerve damage and restore lost or impaired functions. For example, in men with complete spinal cord injury, epidural spinal cord stimulation has enabled the recovery of both ejaculatory reflexes and natural reproduction beyond ejaculation [166]. This discovery is only a preliminary observation; it indicates that current technologies in neuromodulation will greatly benefit men who suffer from infertility due to neurological disease [166].

Genetic editing, such as that of the CRISPR/Cas9 system, mainly works by removing damaged genes and replacing them with healthy ones [162]. Currently, it is experimental in animals and could allow us to understand the genetic causes of male infertility [162]. Eventually, this may help to correct certain infertility problems in men [162]. Safety and ethical issues must be carefully considered before these technologies can be used clinically. Future studies will need to fill these gaps and ensure that these treatments for male infertility are not only safe but also beneficial, accessible, and affordable.

9. Conclusion

In summary, congenital anomalies of the upper and lower urinary tract as well as neuro-urological conditions can affect male sexual function and fertility. Early diagnosis and prompt treatment can contribute significantly to preserving sexual function and fertility as well as quality of life. Progress in surgical techniques and ART has improved patient outcomes. However, it is still essential that the physician treat each patient on the basis of their specific anatomical presentations and clinical history. For lower urinary tract malformations that typically involve the bladder, a broad program of reconstruction combined with fertility preservation measures is essential. Structured care provided by a multidisciplinary team is necessary if one wants to have both the defects repaired and the fertility issue resolved. Anatomical anomalies such as hypospadias, diphallus, or undescended testis directly affect the fertility and sexual function of those affected. Early corrective surgery followed by continuous monitoring into adulthood yields the best results.

For neurogenic patients with multiple sclerosis, spinal cord injuries and CVAs, and in other neurogenic populations such as those born with spinal dysraphisms, sexual dysfunction and infertility challenges pose a complex problem, not just from a physiological dimension alone, but also a psychological one. A coordinated and integrated treatment plan that combines drug therapies with ART and supportive care programs is important for improving sexual performance, fertility results and the overall quality of life of the patient. Personalized nutrition and lifestyle changes provide important support for male fertility. Extensive research is yet lacking and lagging in these fields for the betterment of the male productive health in these patient populations.

Acknowledgements

Published on behalf of the *Kuwait Functional Urology Group*.

Author details

Talal A. Alenezi[1], Abdulrahman Almazeedi[2], Maryam Albuloushi[1], Ali Almoumen[1], Naser Al-Soudan Al-Anazi[3,4], Abdullatif E. Al-Terki[3], Tariq F. Al-Shaiji[2,5] and Said M. Yaiesh[2,5]*

1 Kuwait Board of Urology, Kuwait Institute for Medical Specializations, Kuwait City, Kuwait

2 Urology Unit, Department of Surgery, Jaber Al Ahmad Al Jaber Al Subah Hospital, Kuwait City, Kuwait

3 Urology Unit, Department of Surgery, Al Amiri Hospital, Kuwait City, Kuwait

4 Pediatric Urology Unit, Department of Surgery, Sabah Al Ahmad Urology Center, Kuwait City, Kuwait

5 Kuwait Functional Urology Group, Kuwait

*Address all correspondence to: syaiesh@hotmail.com

References

[1] Kagan M, Pleniceanu O, Vivante A. The genetic basis of congenital anomalies of the kidney and urinary tract. Pediatric Nephrology. 2022;**37**(10):2231-2243. DOI: 10.1007/s00467-021-05420-1

[2] Punjani N, Lamb DJ. Male infertility and genitourinary birth defects: There is more than meets the eye. Fertility and Sterility. 2020;**114**(2):209-218. DOI: 10.1016/j.fertnstert.2020.06.042

[3] Trofimenko V, Brant WO. Fertility and sexual dysfunction issues in adults with genitourinary congenital anomalies. Current Opinion in Urology. 2016;**26**(4):357-362. DOI: 10.1097/MOU.0000000000000295

[4] Campetella M, Marino F, Gavi F, Gandi C, Ragonese M, Coluzzi S, et al. Classification and management of sexual dysfunctions in multiple sclerosis patients: A review of current literature. Urologia. 2023;**90**(4):605-610. DOI: 10.1177/03915603231183751

[5] Delaney KE, Donovan J. Multiple sclerosis and sexual dysfunction: A need for further education and interdisciplinary care. NeuroRehabilitation. 2017;**41**(2):317-329. DOI: 10.3233/NRE-172200

[6] Anderson KD. Targeting recovery: Priorities of the spinal cord-injured population. Journal of Neurotrauma. 2004;**21**(10):1371-1383. DOI: 10.1089/neu.2004.21.1371

[7] Park JH, Ovbiagele B, Feng W. Stroke and sexual dysfunction - A narrative review. Journal of the Neurological Sciences. 2015;**350**(1-2):7-13. DOI: 10.1016/j.jns.2015.02.001

[8] Dudek RW. Embryology. Philadelphia (PA), USA: Wolters Kluwer Health; 2014

[9] Rehman S, Ahmed D. Embryology, Kidney, Bladder, and Ureter. Treasure Island (FL): StatPearls; 2025

[10] Stonebrook E, Hoff M, Spencer JD. Congenital anomalies of the kidney and urinary tract: A clinical review. Current Treatment Options in Pediatrics. 2019;**5**(3):223-235. DOI: 10.1007/s40746-019-00166-3

[11] Mahmoud AH, Talaat IM, Tlili A, Hamoudi R. Congenital anomalies of the kidney and urinary tract. Frontiers in Medicine (Lausanne). 2024;**11**:1384676. DOI: 10.3389/fmed.2024.1384676

[12] Brockwell M, Hergenrother S, Satariano M, Shah R, Raina R. Pathophysiology of congenital anomalies of the kidney and urinary tract: A comprehensive review. Cells. 2024;**13**(22):1866. DOI: 10.3390/cells13221866

[13] Shish L, Reardon E, Kogan S. Fertility prospects for the prune-belly patient: A scoping review. Journal of Pediatric Urology. 2024;**20**(3):446-454. DOI: 10.1016/j.jpurol.2024.01.005

[14] Walawender L, Becknell B, Matsell DG. Congenital anomalies of the kidney and urinary tract: Defining risk factors of disease progression and determinants of outcomes. Pediatric Nephrology. 2023;**38**(12):3963-3973. DOI: 10.1007/s00467-023-05899-w

[15] Capone V, Persico N, Berrettini A, Decramer S, De Marco EA, De Palma D, et al. Definition, diagnosis and management of fetal lower urinary tract obstruction: Consensus of the ERKNet CAKUT-obstructive uropathy work group. Nature Reviews. Urology.

2022;**19**(5):295-303. DOI: 10.1038/s41585-022-00563-8

[16] Palmer BF. Outcomes associated with hypogonadism in men with chronic kidney disease. Advances in Chronic Kidney Disease. 2004;**11**(4):342-347

[17] Chevalier RL. CAKUT: A pediatric and evolutionary perspective on the leading cause of CKD in childhood. Pediatric Reports. 2023;**15**(1):143-153. DOI: 10.3390/pediatric15010012

[18] Lange-Sperandio B, Anders HJ, Stehr M, Chevalier RL, Klaus R. Congenital anomalies of the kidney and urinary tract: A continuum of care. Seminars in Nephrology. 2023;**43**(4):151433. DOI: 10.1016/j.semnephrol.2023.151433

[19] Mitchel MW, Moreno-De-Luca D, Myers SM, Levy RV, Turner S, Ledbetter DH, et al. 17q12 recurrent deletion syndrome. In: Adam MP, Feldman J, Mirzaa GM, Pagon RA, Wallace SE, Amemiya A, editors. GeneReviews. Seattle (WA): GeneReviews((R)); 1993

[20] Hua Tan CS, Ang SF, Yeoh E, Goh BX, Loh WJ, Shum CF, et al. MODY5 hepatocyte nuclear factor 1ss (HNF1ss)-associated nephropathy: Experience from a regional monogenic diabetes referral Centre in Singapore. Journal of Investigative Medicine High Impact Case Reports. 2022;**10**:23247096211065626. DOI: 10.1177/23247096211065626

[21] Alan WP. Campbell Walsh Wein Urology. Philadelphia (PA), USA: Elsevier; 2021. 2 p

[22] Han H, Li J, Lei H, Yin H, Tian L. Microvascular doppler-assisted microsurgical left spermatic-inferior epigastric vein anastomosis for treating nutcracker syndrome-associated varicocele. European Urology Open Science. 2023;**52**:145-152. DOI: 10.1016/j.euros.2023.04.012

[23] Kojo K, Kim J, Saida T, Ohta T, Sano K, Kandori S, et al. Practical step-by-step SYNAPSE VINCENT rendering of three-dimensional graphics in horseshoe kidney with bilateral varicoceles. The JMA Journal. 2024;**7**(4):471-486. DOI: 10.31662/jmaj.2024-0058

[24] Meng J, Xu Y, Shen X, Liang C. A novel frameshift PKD1 mutation in a Chinese patient with autosomal dominant polycystic kidney disease and azoospermia: A case report. Experimental and Therapeutic Medicine. 2019;**17**(1):507-511. DOI: 10.3892/etm.2018.6946

[25] Avellino GJ, Lipshultz LI, Sigman M, Hwang K. Transurethral resection of the ejaculatory ducts: Etiology of obstruction and surgical treatment options. Fertility and Sterility. 2019;**111**(3):427-443. DOI: 10.1016/j.fertnstert.2019.01.001

[26] Glenn JF. Agenesis of the bladder. Journal of the American Medical Association. 1959;**169**(17):2016-2018. DOI: 10.1001/jama.1959.73000340001013

[27] Krull CL, Heyns CF, de Klerk DP. Agenesis of the bladder and urethra: A case report. The Journal of Urology. 1988;**140**(4):793-794. DOI: 10.1016/s0022-5347(17)41815-5

[28] Nazer II, Alhashmi G, Sharief SN, Hefni NA, Ibrahim A, El-Desoky SM, et al. A case of urinary bladder agenesis and bilateral ectopic ureters: A case report. BMC Urology. 2018;**18**(1):83. DOI: 10.1186/s12894-018-0396-6

[29] Yahya MH. Bladder agenesis: A systematic review. Cureus.

2023;**15**(9):e45121. DOI: 10.7759/cureus.45121

[30] Jayachandran D, Bythell M, Platt MW, Rankin J. Register based study of bladder exstrophy-epispadias complex: Prevalence, associated anomalies, prenatal diagnosis and survival. The Journal of Urology. 2011;**186**(5):2056-2060. DOI: 10.1016/j.juro.2011.07.022

[31] Dellenmark-Blom M, Sjostrom S, Abrahamsson K, Holmdahl G. Health-related quality of life among children, adolescents, and adults with bladder exstrophy-epispadias complex: A systematic review of the literature and recommendations for future research. Quality of Life Research. 2019;**28**(6):1389-1412. DOI: 10.1007/s11136-019-02119-7

[32] Uludag S, Guralp O, Akbas M, Aydin Y, Sen C, Uludag S. Bladder exstrophy. Fetal and Pediatric Pathology. 2012;**31**(4):225-229. DOI: 10.3109/15513815.2011.650286

[33] Baumgartner TS, Lue KM, Sirisreetreerux P, Metzger S, Everett RG, Reddy SS, et al. Long-term sexual health outcomes in men with classic bladder exstrophy. BJU International. 2017;**120**(3):422-427. DOI: 10.1111/bju.13866

[34] Reynaud N, Courtois F, Mouriquand P, Morel-Journel N, Charvier K, Gerard M, et al. Male sexuality, fertility, and urinary continence in bladder exstrophy-epispadias complex. The Journal of Sexual Medicine. 2018;**15**(3):314-323. DOI: 10.1016/j.jsxm.2018.01.004

[35] Wheatley JM, Stephens FD, Hutson JM. Prune-belly syndrome: Ongoing controversies regarding pathogenesis and management. Seminars in Pediatric Surgery. 1996;**5**(2):95-106

[36] Arlen AM. Prune belly syndrome: Current perspectives. Pediatric Health, Medicine and Therapeutics. 2019;**10**:75-81

[37] Stephens FD, Gupta D. Pathogenesis of the prune belly syndrome. The Journal of Urology. 1994;**152**(6 Pt 2):2328-2331. DOI: 10.1016/s0022-5347(17)31669-5

[38] Favorito LA, Costa SF, Costa WS, Vieiralves R, Bernardo FO, Sampaio FJB. Study of testicular structure in fetuses with prune belly syndrome. Advances in Urology. 2017;**2017**:3254980. DOI: 10.1155/2017/3254980

[39] Kolettis PN, Ross JH, Kay R, Thomas AJ Jr. Sperm retrieval and intracytoplasmic sperm injection in patients with prune-belly syndrome. Fertility and Sterility. 1999;**72**(5):948-949. DOI: 10.1016/s0015-0282(99)00388-x

[40] Sinatti C, Wolff D, Buncamper M, Verla W, Claes K, Lumen N, et al. Phalloplasty in biological men with penile insufficiency. Journal of Pediatric Urology. 2020;**16**(3):404-405. DOI: 10.1016/j.jpurol.2020.04.015

[41] D'Hauwers KW, Feitz WF, Kremer JA. Bladder exstrophy and male fertility: Pregnancies after ICSI with ejaculated or epididymal sperm. Fertility and Sterility. 2008;**89**(2):387-389. DOI: 10.1016/j.fertnstert.2007.03.005

[42] Pathak P, Ring JD, Delfino KR, Dynda DI, Mathews RI. Complete primary repair of bladder exstrophy: A systematic review. Journal of Pediatric Urology. 2020;**16**(2):149-153. DOI: 10.1016/j.jpurol.2020.01.004

[43] Berrettini A, Sampogna G, Gnech M, Montanari E, Manzoni G, Di Grazia M, et al. Substitution phalloplasty in patients with bladder exstrophy-epispadias

complex: A systematic review of techniques, complications and outcomes. The Journal of Sexual Medicine. 2021;**18**(2):400-409. DOI: 10.1016/j.jsxm.2020.10.007

[44] Haddad E, Hayes LC, Price D, Vallery CG, Somers M, Borer JG. Ensuring our exstrophy-epispadias complex patients and families thrive. Pediatric Nephrology. 2024;**39**(2):371-382. DOI: 10.1007/s00467-023-06049-y

[45] Donaire AE, Mendez MD. Hypospadias. In: StatPearls. Treasure Island (FL): StatPearls; 2025

[46] Leslie SW, Sajjad H, Villanueva CA. Cryptorchidism. In: StatPearls. Florida (FL), USA: Treasure Island (FL); 2025

[47] Rodriguez Fernandez V, Lopez Ramon YCC, Marin Ortiz E, Sarmiento CN. Accurate diagnosis of severe hypospadias using 2D and 3D ultrasounds. Case Reports in Obstetrics and Gynecology. 2016;**2016**:2450341. DOI: 10.1155/2016/2450341

[48] Effendi R, Situmorang GR, Wahyudi I, Rodjani A, Raharja PAR, Abbas TO. Adult sexual function following hypospadias repair in childhood: A systematic review and meta-analysis of long-term patient outcomes. Urology. 2025. DOI: 10.1016/j.urology.2025.05.015 [Online ahead of print]

[49] Mirshemirani AR, Sadeghyian N, Mohajerzadeh L, Molayee H, Ghaffari P. Diphallus: Report on six cases and review of the literature. Iranian Journal of Pediatrics. 2010;**20**(3):353-357

[50] Keays MA, Dave S. Current hypospadias management: Diagnosis, surgical management, and long-term patient-centred outcomes. Canadian Urological Association Journal. 2017;**11**(1-2Suppl1):S48-S53. DOI: 10.5489/cuaj.4386

[51] Bocchino AC, Cocci A, Pezzoli M, Elia A, Landi L, Mantovani A, et al. Long-term functional, sexual, and cosmetic outcomes in adult patients who underwent hypospadias repair during childhood at a highly specialized Italian pediatric hospital. Urology Research and Practice. 2024;**50**(2):127-133. DOI: 10.5152/tud.2024.24005

[52] Mutlu N, Baykal M, Merder E, Culha M, Canbazoglu N. Diphallus with urethral duplications. International Urology and Nephrology. 1999;**31**(2):253-255. DOI: 10.1023/a:1007141228452

[53] Messerlian C, Zhang Y, Sun Y, Wang Y, Mustieles V. An ounce of prevention is worth a pound of cure: Time to focus on preconception workplace reproductive health. Human Reproduction. 2021;**37**(1):1-4. DOI: 10.1093/humrep/deab263

[54] Lammers RJM, Tsachouridis G, Andersson MK, Dormeus S, Ekerhult TO, Frankiewicz M, et al. What should be next in lifelong posterior hypospadias: Conclusions from the 2023 ERN eUROGEN and EJP-RD networking meeting. Neurourology and Urodynamics. 2024;**43**(5):1097-1103. DOI: 10.1002/nau.25305

[55] Van Steirteghem A, Devroey P, Liebaers I. Intracytoplasmic sperm injection. Molecular and Cellular Endocrinology. 2002;**186**(2):199-203. DOI: 10.1016/s0303-7207(01)00658-x

[56] Kenney LB, Antal Z, Ginsberg JP, Hoppe BS, Bober SL, Yu RN, et al. Improving male reproductive health after childhood, adolescent, and young adult cancer: Progress and future directions for

survivorship research. Journal of Clinical Oncology. 2018;**36**(21):2160-2168. DOI: 10.1200/JCO.2017.76.3839

[57] Pahlavan F, Niknejad F, Sajadi H, Vosough A. Unilateral kidney agenesis and other kidney anomalies in infertile men with congenital bilateral absence of vas deferens: A cross-sectional study. International Journal of Fertility and Sterility. 2022;**16**(3):152-155. DOI: 10.22074/ijfs.2021.535148.1166

[58] Zheng L, Wang L, Jiang H, Jiang T. Azoospermia due to functional and partial ejaculatory duct obstruction: A rare case report and literature review. American Journal of Men's Health. 2024;**18**(5):15579883241281668. DOI: 10.1177/15579883241281668

[59] Cai H, Qing X, Niringiyumukiza JD, Zhan X, Mo D, Zhou Y, et al. CFTR variants and renal abnormalities in males with congenital unilateral absence of the vas deferens (CUAVD): A systematic review and meta-analysis of observational studies. Genetics in Medicine. 2019;**21**(4):826-836. DOI: 10.1038/s41436-018-0262-7

[60] Kumar S, Ki G, Khalil-Khan A, ADP AP, Sathiamoorthy R, Raju E. Zinner syndrome. Cureus. 2022;**14**(11):e31308. DOI: 10.7759/cureus.31308

[61] Acien P, Acien M. Renal agenesis, associated genital malformations, and responsible genes. Fertility and Sterility. 2021;**116**(5):1370-1371. DOI: 10.1016/j.fertnstert.2021.08.042

[62] Sawaftah Z, Sawafta K, Hattab M, Rub AAA, Sawafta O, Khamaysa J, et al. Zinner syndrome unveiled: Ectopic ureter and seminal vesicle cyst leading to urinary dysfunction: A case report. Radiology Case Reports. 2025;**20**(3):1721-1725. DOI: 10.1016/j.radcr.2024.12.017

[63] Hofmann A, Vauth F, Roesch WH. Zinner syndrome and infertility horizontal line a literature review based on a clinical case. International Journal of Impotence Research. 2021;**33**(2):191-195. DOI: 10.1038/s41443-020-00360-0

[64] Zhou YH, Dong JJ, Zhi EL, Yao CC, Huang YH, Tian RH, et al. Clinical features and microsurgical reconstruction of congenital unilateral absence of the vas deferens with obstructive azoospermia: A tertiary care center experience. Asian Journal of Andrology. 2023;**25**(1):73-77. DOI: 10.4103/aja20225

[65] Cai Z, Li H. Congenital bilateral absence of the vas deferens. Frontiers in Genetics. 2022;**13**:775123. DOI: 10.3389/fgene.2022.775123

[66] Achermann APP, Esteves SC. Diagnosis and management of infertility due to ejaculatory duct obstruction: Summary evidence. International Braz J Urol. 2021;**47**(4):868-881. DOI: 10.1590/S1677-5538.IBJU.2020.0536

[67] Chiang GCM. In: Pun, editor. Disorders of the Penis and Scrotum. Philadelphia (PA), USA: Saunders Elsevier; 2010. pp. 467-483

[68] Khatwa UA, Menon PS. Management of undescended testis. Indian Journal of Pediatrics. 2000;**67**(6):449-454. DOI: 10.1007/BF02859466

[69] Shin J, Jeon GW. Comparison of diagnostic and treatment guidelines for undescended testis. Clinical and Experimental Pediatrics. 2020;**63**(11):415-421. DOI: 10.3345/cep.2019.01438

[70] Pakkasjarvi N, Taskinen S. Surgical treatment of cryptorchidism: Current insights and future directions. Frontiers in Endocrinology (Lausanne).

2024;**15**:1327957. DOI: 10.3389/fendo.2024.1327957

[71] van Brakel J, Kranse R, de Muinck Keizer-Schrama SM, Hendriks AE, de Jong FH, Hack WW, et al. Fertility potential in a cohort of 65 men with previously acquired undescended testes. Journal of Pediatric Surgery. 2014;**49**(4):599-605. DOI: 10.1016/j.jpedsurg.2013.09.020

[72] Lee PA, Houk CP. Cryptorchidism. Current Opinion in Endocrinology, Diabetes, and Obesity. 2013;**20**(3):210-216. DOI: 10.1097/MED.0b013e32835ffc7d

[73] BSR A, Dumann E, Fawkner-Corbett D, Kwok C, Skerritt C, Paediatric Surgery Trainees Research N. Systematic review and meta-analysis comparing outcomes following orchidopexy for cryptorchidism before or after 1 year of age. BJS Open. 2018;**2**(1):1-12. DOI: 10.1002/bjs5.36

[74] Hadziselimovic F, Herzog B. Treatment with a luteinizing hormone-releasing hormone analogue after successful orchiopexy markedly improves the chance of fertility later in life. The Journal of Urology. 1997;**158**(3 Pt 2):1193-1195. DOI: 10.1097/00005392-199709000-00130

[75] Wood HM, Elder JS. Cryptorchidism and testicular cancer: Separating fact from fiction. The Journal of Urology. 2009;**181**(2):452-461. DOI: 10.1016/j.juro.2008.10.074

[76] Lee PA, O'Leary LA, Songer NJ, Coughlin MT, Bellinger MF, LaPorte RE. Paternity after bilateral cryptorchidism. A controlled study. Archives of Pediatrics and Adolescent Medicine. 1997;**151**(3):260-263. DOI: 10.1001/archpedi.1997.02170400046008

[77] Hadziselimovic F, Hoecht B. Testicular histology related to fertility outcome and postpubertal hormone status in cryptorchidism. Klinische Pädiatrie. 2008;**220**(5):302-307. DOI: 10.1055/s-2007-993194

[78] Fan L, Shi L, Liu S, Zhang Z, Shi J. Bilateral versus unilateral orchidopexy: IVF/ICSI-ET outcomes. Frontiers in Endocrinology (Lausanne). 2024;**15**:1294884. DOI: 10.3389/fendo.2024.1294884

[79] Kim SW, Lee J, Lee TH, Kim DS, Song SH, Kim DK. Azoospermic men with a history of cryptorchidism treated by orchiopexy have favorable outcomes after testicular sperm extraction: A systematic review and meta-analysis. The World Journal of Men's Health. 2023;**41**(1):81-93. DOI: 10.5534/wjmh.210198

[80] Moussaoui D, Surbone A, Adam C, Diesch-Furlanetto T, Girardin C, Benard J, et al. Testicular tissue cryopreservation for fertility preservation in prepubertal and adolescent boys: A 6 year experience from a Swiss multi-center network. Frontiers in Pediatrics. 2022;**10**:909000. DOI: 10.3389/fped.2022.909000

[81] Kolon TF, Herndon CD, Baker LA, Baskin LS, Baxter CG, Cheng EY, et al. Evaluation and treatment of cryptorchidism: AUA guideline. The Journal of Urology. 2014;**192**(2):337-345. DOI: 10.1016/j.juro.2014.05.005

[82] Banks K, Tuazon E, Berhane K, Koh CJ, De Filippo RE, Chang A, et al. Cryptorchidism and testicular germ cell tumors: Comprehensive meta-analysis reveals that association between these conditions diminished over time and is modified by clinical characteristics. Frontiers in Endocrinology (Lausanne). 2012;**3**:182. DOI: 10.3389/fendo.2012.00182

[83] Dighriri IM, Aldalbahi AA, Albeladi F, Tahiri AA, Kinani EM,

Almohsen RA, et al. An overview of the history, pathophysiology, and pharmacological interventions of multiple sclerosis. Cureus. 2023;**15**(1):e33242. DOI: 10.7759/cureus.33242

[84] Geng H, Ye Q, Lin X, Simpson-Yap S, Zhou Y, Tang D. Impact of multiple sclerosis on male sexual and reproductive health. Multiple Sclerosis and Related Disorders. 2023;**79**:105059. DOI: 10.1016/j.msard.2023.105059

[85] Toljan K, Briggs FBS. Male sexual and reproductive health in multiple sclerosis: A scoping review. Journal of Neurology. 2024;**271**(5):2169-2181. DOI: 10.1007/s00415-024-12250-2

[86] Redelman MJ. Sexual difficulties for persons with multiple sclerosis in New South Wales, Australia. International Journal of Rehabilitation Research. 2009;**32**(4):337-347. DOI: 10.1097/MRR.0b013e3283298166

[87] Dastoorpoor M, Zamanian M, Moradzadeh R, Nabavi SM, Kousari R. Prevalence of sexual dysfunction in men with multiple sclerosis: A systematic review and meta-analysis. Systematic Reviews. 2021;**10**(1):10. DOI: 10.1186/s13643-020-01560-x

[88] DasGupta R, Fowler CJ. Bladder, bowel and sexual dysfunction in multiple sclerosis: Management strategies. Drugs. 2003;**63**(2):153-166. DOI: 10.2165/00003495-200363020-00003

[89] Massarotti C, Sbragia E, Gazzo I, Stigliani S, Inglese M, Anserini P. Effect of multiple sclerosis and its treatments on male fertility: Cues for future research. Journal of Clinical Medicine. 2021;**10**(22):5401. DOI: 10.3390/jcm10225401

[90] Guo ZN, He SY, Zhang HL, Wu J, Yang Y. Multiple sclerosis and sexual dysfunction. Asian Journal of Andrology. 2012;**14**(4):530-535. DOI: 10.1038/aja.2011.110

[91] Shaygannejad V, Mirmosayyeb O, Vaheb S, Nehzat N, Ghajarzadeh M. The prevalence of sexual dysfunction and erectile dysfunction in men with multiple sclerosis: A systematic review and meta-analysis. Neurologia (England Ed). 2025;**40**(1):22-31. DOI: 10.1016/j.nrleng.2022.08.002

[92] Lima R, Monteiro A, Salgado AJ, Monteiro S, Silva NA. Pathophysiology and therapeutic approaches for spinal cord injury. International Journal of Molecular Sciences. 2022;**23**(22):13833. DOI: 10.3390/ijms232213833

[93] Anderson R, Moses R, Lenherr S, Hotaling JM, Myers J. Spinal cord injury and male infertility-a review of current literature, knowledge gaps, and future research. The Translational Andrology and **Urology**. 2018;**7**(Suppl. 3):S373-SS82. DOI: 10.21037/tau.2018.04.12

[94] Ibrahim E. Penile vibratory stimulation in men with spinal cord injury: An educational video demonstration. Fertility and Sterility. 2024;**121**(3):545-547. DOI: 10.1016/j.fertnstert.2023.12.013

[95] Lombardi G, Macchiarella A, Cecconi F, Del Popolo G. Ten-year follow-up of sildenafil use in spinal cord-injured patients with erectile dysfunction. The Journal of Sexual Medicine. 2009;**6**(12):3449-3457. DOI: 10.1111/j.1743-6109.2009.01426.x

[96] Pacheco, de Melo K, Siqueira S, de Souza G, Ibrahim E, Lynne CM, Brackett NL, et al. Spinal cord injury and male infertility: Effect of the inflammasome proteins on semen quality. The Journal of

Spinal Cord Medicine. 2025:1-7. DOI: 10.1080/10790268.2025.2472095 [Online ahead of print]

[97] Di Bello F, Creta M, Napolitano L, Califano G, Passaro F, Morra S, et al. Male sexual dysfunction and infertility in spinal cord injury patients: State-of-the-art and future perspectives. Journal of Personalized Medicine. 2022;**12**(6):873. DOI: 10.3390/jpm12060873

[98] Khaku AS, Tadi P. Cerebrovascular disease. In: StatPearls. Treasure Island (FL): StatPearls; 2025

[99] Zhu Y, Xin X, Yu Z, Guan S, Wang J, Liu Q, et al. Causal associations of male infertility with stroke: A two-sample Mendelian randomization study. Frontiers in Endocrinology (Lausanne). 2024;**15**:1338077. DOI: 10.3389/fendo.2024.1338077

[100] Contrada M, Cerasa A, Pucci C, Ciancarelli I, Pioggia G, Tonin P, et al. Talking about sexuality in stroke individuals: The new era of sexual rehabilitation. Journal of Clinical Medicine. 2023;**12**(12):3988. DOI: 10.3390/jcm12123988

[101] Calabro RS. Post-stroke sexual dysfunction in men: Epidemiology, diagnostic work-up, and treatment. Innovations in Clinical Neuroscience. 2022;**19**(7-9):12-16

[102] Schjorring CB, Eddelien HS, Butt JH, Kruuse C. High prevalence of erectile dysfunction in male patients with acute stroke was associated with age but not to modifiable cardiovascular risk factors. BMJ Neurology Open. 2024;**6**(2):e000795. DOI: 10.1136/bmjno-2024-000795

[103] Montalvan V, Ulrich AK, Tirschwell DL, Zunt JR. Assessing sexual dysfunction among stroke survivors and barriers to address this issue by physicians at a Latin American reference hospital. Clinical Neurology and Neurosurgery. 2021;**205**:106642. DOI: 10.1016/j.clineuro.2021.106642

[104] Vikan JK, Nilsson MI, Bushnik T, Deng W, Elessi K, Frost-Bareket Y, et al. Sexual health policies in stroke rehabilitation: A multi national study. Journal of Rehabilitation Medicine. 2019;**51**(5):361-368. DOI: 10.2340/16501977-2552

[105] Cong R, Zhang Q, Wang Y, Meng X, Wang Z, Song N. Two cases of psychogenic anejaculation patients got normal ejaculation ability after penile vibratory stimulation or electroejaculation. The Translational Andrology and Urology. 2019;**8**(6):758-761. DOI: 10.21037/tau.2019.10.11

[106] Rhoden EL, Teloken C, Sogari PR, Vargas Souto CA. The use of the simplified international index of erectile function (IIEF-5) as a diagnostic tool to study the prevalence of erectile dysfunction. International Journal of Impotence Research. 2002;**14**(4):245-250. DOI: 10.1038/sj.ijir.3900859

[107] Huang SA, Lie JD. Phosphodiesterase-5 (PDE5) inhibitors In the management of erectile dysfunction. P T. 2013;**38**(7):407-419

[108] Aikman K, Oliffe JL, Kelly MT, McCuaig F. Sexual health in men with traumatic spinal cord injuries: A review and recommendations for primary health-care providers. American Journal of Men's Health. 2018;**12**(6):2044-2054. DOI: 10.1177/1557988318790883

[109] Cissen M, Bensdorp A, Cohlen BJ, Repping S, de Bruin JP, van Wely M. Assisted reproductive technologies for male subfertility. Cochrane Database of Systematic

Reviews. 2016;**2**(2):CD000360. DOI: 10.1002/14651858.CD000360.pub5

[110] Rague JT, Hirsch J, Meyer T, Streur C, Rosoklija I, Kielb S, et al. Perspectives of young men with spina bifida on fertility potential and future parenthood. Urology. 2025;**195**:66-73. DOI: 10.1016/j.urology.2024.09.012

[111] Moussa M, Papatsoris AG, Chakra MA, Fares Y, Dabboucy B, Dellis A. Perspectives on urological care in spina bifida patients. Intractable and Rare Diseases Research. 2021;**10**(1):1-10. DOI: 10.5582/irdr.2020.03077

[112] Venkataramana NK. Spinal dysraphism. Journal of Pediatric Neurosciences. 2011;**6**(Suppl. 1):S31-S40. DOI: 10.4103/1817-1745.85707

[113] Chellathurai A, Kathirvelu G, Mukkada PJ, Rajendran K, Ramani R. Spinal dysraphisms: A new anatomical-clinicoradiological classification. Indian Journal of Radiology and Imaging. 2021;**31**(4):809-829. DOI: 10.1055/s-0041-1741100

[114] Cass AS, Bloom BA, Luxenberg M. Sexual function in adults with myelomeningocele. The Journal of Urology. 1986;**136**(2):425-426. DOI: 10.1016/s0022-5347(17)44891-9

[115] Bomalaski MD, Teague JL, Brooks B. The long-term impact of urological management on the quality of life of children with spina bifida. The Journal of Urology. 1995;**154**(2 Pt 2):778-781. DOI: 10.1097/00005392-199508000-00120

[116] Hultling C, Levi R, Amark SP, Sjoblom P. Semen retrieval and analysis in men with myelomeningocele. Developmental Medicine and Child Neurology. 2000;**42**(10):681-684. DOI: 10.1017/s0012162200001250

[117] Conti CR, Pepine CJ, Sweeney M. Efficacy and safety of sildenafil citrate in the treatment of erectile dysfunction in patients with ischemic heart disease. The American Journal of Cardiology. 1999;**83**(5A):29C-34C. DOI: 10.1016/s0002-9149(99)00045-4

[118] Deng N, Thirumavalavan N, Beilan JA, Tatem AJ, Hockenberry MS, Pastuszak AW, et al. Sexual dysfunction and infertility in the male spina bifida patient. The Translational Andrology and Urology. 2018;**7**(6):941-949. DOI: 10.21037/tau.2018.10.08

[119] Reilly J, Oates R. Preliminary investigation of the potential fertility status of postpubertal males with myelodysplasia. The Journal of Urology. 1992;**147**(Suppl.):75A

[120] Palmer JS, Kaplan WE, Firlit CF. Erectile dysfunction in patients with spina bifida is a treatable condition. The Journal of Urology. 2000;**164**(3 Pt 2):958-961. DOI: 10.1097/00005392-200009020-00009

[121] Vanderhout SM, Rastegar Panah M, Garcia-Bailo B, Grace-Farfaglia P, Samsel K, Dockray J, et al. Nutrition, genetic variation and male fertility. The Translational Andrology and Urology. 2021;**10**(3):1410-1431. DOI: 10.21037/tau-20-592

[122] Monteiro J, Bicho M, Valente A. The contribution of precision nutrition intervention in subfertile couples. Nutrients. 2024;**17**(1):103. DOI: 10.3390/nu17010103

[123] Tesarik J. Lifestyle and environmental factors affecting male fertility, individual predisposition, prevention, and intervention. International Journal of Molecular Sciences. 2025;**26**(6):2797. DOI: 10.3390/ijms26062797

[124] Tully CA, Alesi S, McPherson NO, Sharkey DJ, Teong XT, Tay CT, et al. Assessing the influence of preconception diet on male fertility: A systematic scoping review. Human Reproduction Update. 2024;**30**(3):243-261. DOI: 10.1093/humupd/dmad035

[125] Song W, Peng Y, Jiang Z, Quan Z. Effectiveness of exercise interventions on sperm quality: A systematic review and network meta-analysis. Frontiers in Endocrinology (Lausanne). 2025;**16**:1537271. DOI: 10.3389/fendo.2025.1537271

[126] Torkel S, Wang R, Norman RJ, Zhao L, Liu K, Boden D, et al. Barriers and enablers to a healthy lifestyle in people with infertility: A mixed-methods systematic review. Human Reproduction Update. 2024;**30**(5):569-583. DOI: 10.1093/humupd/dmae011

[127] Heston AL, Esmonde NO, Dugi DD 3rd, Berli JU. Phalloplasty: Techniques and outcomes. The Translational Andrology and Urology. 2019;**8**(3):254-265. DOI: 10.21037/tau.2019.05.05

[128] Morrison SD, Shakir A, Vyas KS, Kirby J, Crane CN, Lee GK. Phalloplasty: A review of techniques and outcomes. Plastic and Reconstructive Surgery. 2016;**138**(3):594-615. DOI: 10.1097/PRS.0000000000002518

[129] Demirtas G, Tagcı S, Yayla D, Ergani HM, Ekberli G, Karabulut B, et al. Phalloplasty in children with severe penile tissue loss: Single center case series. Medicina. 2025;**61**(7):1124

[130] Harris TGW, Khandge P, Wu WJ, Leto Barone AA, Manyevitch R, Sholklapper T, et al. Sexual health outcomes after penile reconstruction in the exstrophy-epispadias complex. Journal of Pediatric Urology. 2022;**18**(6):747-755. DOI: 10.1016/j.jpurol.2022.02.016

[131] Pang KH, Muneer A, Alnajjar HM. A systematic review of penile prosthesis insertion in patients with spinal cord injury. Sexual Medicine Reviews. 2022;**10**(3):468-477. DOI: 10.1016/j.sxmr.2022.01.004

[132] Town MV, Kim KJ, Vu A, Haffar A, Morganstern BA. Bladder exstrophy: Navigating long-term outcomes. The Translational Andrology and Urology. 2025;**14**(6):1797-1806. DOI: 10.21037/tau-2024-631

[133] Nerli RB, Shirol SS, Guntaka A, Patil S, Hiremath MB. Genital reconstruction in exstrophy patients. Indian Journal of Urology. 2012;**28**(3):280-285. DOI: 10.4103/0970-1591.102701

[134] Ricketts S, Hunter-Smith DJ, Coombs CJ. Quality of life after penile reconstruction using the radial forearm flap in adult bladder exstrophy patients - Technique and outcomes. ANZ Journal of Surgery. 2011;**81**(1-2):52-55. DOI: 10.1111/j.1445-2197.2010.05482.x

[135] Wilson CJ, Pistrang N, Woodhouse CR, Christie D. The psychosocial impact of bladder exstrophy in adolescence. The Journal of Adolescent Health. 2007;**41**(5):504-508. DOI: 10.1016/j.jadohealth.2007.05.021

[136] Sinha V, Elliott S, Ibrahim E, Lynne CM, Brackett NL. Reproductive health of men with spinal cord injury. Topics in Spinal Cord Injury Rehabilitation (TSCIR). 2017;**23**(1):31-41. DOI: 10.1310/sci2301-31

[137] Brackett NL. Infertility in men with spinal cord injury: Research and treatment. Scientifica

(Cairo). 2012;**2012**:578257. DOI: 10.6064/2012/578257

[138] Yaiesh S, Hopkins DT, Perera S, Webb N, Elmer S. Transition adolescent functional urology in 2024: Current challenges and into the future. Current Bladder Dysfunction Reports. 2024;**19**(3):245-250. DOI: 10.1007/s11884-024-00754-6

[139] Wood D. Adolescent urology: Developing lifelong care for congenital anomalies. Nature Reviews. Urology. 2014;**11**(5):289-296. DOI: 10.1038/nrurol.2014.71

[140] Morlacco A, Bianco M, Dal Moro F. Transitional care in urology: The road to independence. Nature Reviews. Urology. 2022;**19**(12):691-692. DOI: 10.1038/s41585-022-00653-7

[141] Lambert SM. Transitional care in pediatric urology. Seminars in Pediatric Surgery. 2015;**24**(2):73-78. DOI: 10.1053/j.sempedsurg.2015.01.004

[142] Suson KD. Transitional urology for male adolescents: What adult urologists should know. Current Urology Reports. 2016;**17**(10):71. DOI: 10.1007/s11934-016-0630-2

[143] Blubaum A, Lewis J, Frimberger D, Slobodov G. 9-year evaluation of a transitional care program for congenital neurogenic bladder patients. Urology. 2023;**180**:285-290. DOI: 10.1016/j.urology.2023.06.023

[144] Donmez MI, Selvi I, Tantekin A, Oktar T, Ziylan O. Outcomes of a newly established transitional urology outpatient clinic: A real-world experience. International Urology and Nephrology. 2023;**55**(12):3021-3031. DOI: 10.1007/s11255-023-03732-9

[145] Chan R, Scovell J, Jeng Z, Rajanahally S, Boone T, Khavari R. The fate of transitional urology patients referred to a tertiary transitional care center. Urology. 2014;**84**(6):1544-1548. DOI: 10.1016/j.urology.2014.08.022

[146] Leslie SW, Soon-Sutton TL, Khan MAB. Male infertility. In: StatPearls. Treasure Island (FL): StatPearls; 2025

[147] Brackett NL, Lynne CM, Ibrahim E, Ohl DA, Sonksen J. Treatment of infertility in men with spinal cord injury. Nature Reviews. Urology. 2010;**7**(3):162-172. DOI: 10.1038/nrurol.2010.7

[148] Linsenmeyer TA. Treatment of erectile dysfunction following spinal cord injury. Current Urology Reports. 2009;**10**(6):478-484. DOI: 10.1007/s11934-009-0076-x

[149] Fode M, Krogh-Jespersen S, Brackett NL, Ohl DA, Lynne CM, Sonksen J. Male sexual dysfunction and infertility associated with neurological disorders. Asian Journal of Andrology. 2012;**14**(1):61-68. DOI: 10.1038/aja.2011.70

[150] Alexander MS, Aisen CM, Alexander SM, Aisen ML. Sexual concerns after spinal cord injury: An update on management. NeuroRehabilitation. 2017;**41**(2):343-357. DOI: 10.3233/NRE-172202

[151] Anderson KD, Borisoff JF, Johnson RD, Stiens SA, Elliott SL. The impact of spinal cord injury on sexual function: Concerns of the general population. Spinal Cord. 2007;**45**(5):328-337. DOI: 10.1038/sj.sc.3101977

[152] SooHoo M, Baker Z, Do C, Lavoie C, Montano Z, Kysh L, et al. Mental health, psychosocial functioning, and health-related quality of life of children and adolescents with bladder exstrophy,

cloacal exstrophy, and epispadias: A scoping review. Journal of Pediatric Urology. 2024;**20**(6):1044-1056. DOI: 10.1016/j.jpurol.2024.09.013

[153] Nahata L, Quinn GP, Tishelman AC, Section OE. Counseling in pediatric populations at risk for infertility and/or sexual function concerns. Pediatrics. 2018;**142**(2):e20181435. DOI: 10.1542/peds.2018-1435

[154] Senecal K, Thys K, Vears DF, Van Assche K, Knoppers BM, Borry P. Legal approaches regarding health-care decisions involving minors: Implications for next-generation sequencing. European Journal of Human Genetics. 2016;**24**(11):1559-1564. DOI: 10.1038/ejhg.2016.61

[155] Zampieri N. Fertility preservation in pediatric age: Future perspective among andrological diseases. Life (Basel). 2023;**13**(9):193. DOI: 10.3390/life13091934

[156] Dreer LE, Devivo MJ, Novack TA, Krzywanski S, Marson DC. Cognitive predictors of medical decision-making capacity in traumatic brain injury. Rehabilitation Psychology. 2008;**53**(4):486-497. DOI: 10.1037/a0013798

[157] Radmayr CBG, Bujons A, Burgu B, Castagnetti M, t' Hoen LA, O'Kelly F, et al. EAU guidelines on paediatric urology 2025. In: Limited Update April 2025. 2025 update ed. Arnhem, The Netherlands: European Association of Urology; 2025

[158] Braverman AM, Davoudian T, Levin IK, Bocage A, Wodoslawsky S. Depression, anxiety, quality of life, and infertility: A global lens on the last decade of research. Fertility and Sterility. 2024;**121**(3):379-383. DOI: 10.1016/j.fertnstert.2024.01.013

[159] Alirezaei S, Taghipour A, Latifnejad RR. The effect of infertility counseling interventions on marital and sexual satisfaction of infertile couples: A systematic review and meta-analysis. The International Journal of Reproductive BioMedicine. 2022;**20**(10):795-806. DOI: 10.18502/ijrm.v20i10.12264

[160] McCabe MP, Althof SE. A systematic review of the psychosocial outcomes associated with erectile dysfunction: Does the impact of erectile dysfunction extend beyond a man's inability to have sex? The Journal of Sexual Medicine. 2014;**11**(2):347-363. DOI: 10.1111/jsm.12374

[161] Saraf AJ, Nahata L. Fertility counseling and preservation: Considerations for the pediatric endocrinologist. Translational Pediatrics. 2017;**6**(4):313-322. DOI: 10.21037/tp.2017.07.02

[162] Gul M, Russo GI, Kandil H, Boitrelle F, Saleh R, Chung E, et al. Male infertility: New developments, current challenges, and future directions. The World Journal of Men's Health. 2024;**42**(3):502-517. DOI: 10.5534/wjmh.230232

[163] Wu JX, Xia T, She LP, Lin S, Luo XM. Stem cell therapies for human infertility: Advantages and challenges. Cell Transplantation. 2022;**31**:9636897221083252. DOI: 10.1177/09636897221083252

[164] Naik N, Roth B, Lundy SD. Artificial intelligence for clinical management of male infertility, a scoping review. Current Urology Reports. 2024;**26**(1):17. DOI: 10.1007/s11934-024-01239-z

[165] Etafy M, Gudeloglu A, Brahmbhatt JV, Parekattil SJ. Review of the role of robotic surgery in male

infertility. Arab Journal of Urology. 2018;**16**(1):148-156. DOI: 10.1016/j.aju.2017.11.006

[166] Rybka V, Sediva K, Spackova L, Kolar P, Bradac O, Kriz J. Epidural spinal cord stimulation can facilitate ejaculatory response in spinal cord injury individuals: A report of two cases. The International Journal of Neuroscience. 2024;**134**(11):1357-1364. DOI: 10.1080/00207454.2023.2273772

Chapter 4

Emerging Therapies Targeting Male Reproductive Aging Processes

Shabnoor Iqbal and Usman Mir Khan

Abstract

Testicular aging represents a complex biological process characterized by progressive structural and functional decline, leading to diminished testosterone production and impaired reproductive capacity. This phenomenon exerts systemic consequences, contributing to sexual dysfunction, metabolic syndrome, osteoporosis, and neurocognitive impairments. Advanced paternal age further compounds reproductive risks, correlating with increased de novo mutations and elevated incidence of genetic disorders in offspring. Current treatments, including testosterone replacement therapy (TRT), improve bone density and metabolic health but do not fully reverse aging effects. Emerging strategies target inflammation and oxidative stress, with COX-2 inhibitors (e.g., NS398) enhancing testosterone synthesis and antioxidants (e.g., vitamins D, C, E, zinc, and selenium) improving sperm quality. Additionally, novel pharmacotherapies for male sexual dysfunction—such as PDE5 inhibitors (sildenafil, vardenafil), Maxi-K channel activators (NS1619), and nitric oxide donors (L-arginine, MED2005)—show potential in improving erectile function and semen parameters. However, responses vary, and dopamine agonists (e.g., cabergoline) are effective only in hyperprolactinemia-related infertility. Combination therapies integrating hormonal and antioxidant treatments may optimize outcomes, but further research is needed to refine dosing, mechanisms, and long-term safety. A personalized, pathophysiology-driven approach is essential for managing age-related testicular dysfunction and preserving male reproductive health.

Keywords: testicular aging, testosterone decline, male infertility, oxidative stress, PDE5 inhibitors, antioxidant therapy, personalized treatment

1. Introduction

The testes serve dual physiological functions as both endocrine organs and sites of gametogenesis. Their primary endocrine product, testosterone, is synthesized under the regulatory control of the hypothalamic-pituitary-gonadal axis. This steroid hormone exerts systemic effects, influencing cardiovascular physiology, musculoskeletal integrity, metabolic regulation, neurological processes, and reproductive capacity [1]. As men age, their testes undergo significant degenerative changes. These include a decline in testosterone production, a deterioration of the testicular environment, a loss of function in Leydig cells, and reduced efficiency in sperm production [2]. The reduction in testosterone can start at different points throughout adulthood and is linked to a variety of clinical symptoms. These may include metabolic imbalance, sexual dysfunction, decreased bone strength, emotional instability, and memory or cognitive issues—all of which contribute to a decline in overall well-being and quality of life [3]. Research suggests that nearly 20% of men aged 60 and above experience clinically low testosterone levels, with prevalence increasing to about 50% in those over 80 years. On a broader scale, testicular aging affects male fertility rates and shifts in workforce composition, thereby contributing to the economic and social pressures associated with an aging global population [4]. A comprehensive understanding of the complex biological mechanisms underlying testicular aging—including endocrine dysregulation, oxidative stress accumulation, cellular senescence, and microenvironmental alterations—is essential for developing targeted interventions to preserve male reproductive and systemic health in aging populations [5]. Contemporary research is overcoming current therapeutic limitations through innovative approaches combining multi-omics profiling, cellular senescence interventions, and regenerative technologies to develop precision treatments for testicular aging. These advancements address critical demographic challenges posed by aging populations and the systemic health consequences of gonadal dysfunction. The hypothalamic-pituitary-testicular axis undergoes progressive dysregulation with aging, characterized by decreased GnRH pulsatility, reduced pituitary secretion of LH and FSH, and declining Leydig cell responsiveness. These changes lead to impaired testosterone synthesis and spermatogenesis, exacerbated by deteriorating testicular microenvironments and altered sperm proteomes that diminish fertility potential. Concurrently, age-related attenuation of hormonal feedback mechanisms perpetuates endocrine imbalance, contributing to multisystem manifestations, including cardiovascular risk, musculoskeletal deterioration, metabolic dysfunction, and cognitive decline [6, 7].

1.1 Sperm profile, fertility, and age

Aging has been recognized as a contributing factor to reduced fertility in both males and females. While women experience a sharp decline in reproductive capacity between the ages of 35 and 40, the decline in male fertility is generally more gradual. Ford et al. [8] observed that men over 35 years of age had roughly half the adjusted probability of achieving conception within a year, compared to those younger than 25 years, in a study involving untreated couples. Evidence from assisted reproductive techniques, including in vitro fertilization (IVF) and intrauterine insemination (IUI), reveals that increased paternal age correlates with a heightened risk of miscarriage and decreased implantation and pregnancy success rates [9–11]. Even in cycles using donor oocytes—where maternal age is standardized—advanced paternal age has been linked to diminished fertilization rates, reduced embryo quality, and lower chances of live birth [12–14]. These observations imply that aging in males may compromise sperm fertilization capacity and the ability to support healthy embryonic development [15]. However, the extent to which conventional semen parameters—such as sperm count, motility, and morphology—are affected by age remains contentious, with some studies reporting significant deterioration, while others find minimal or no change [16–18]. A potential reason for this discrepancy is variation in ejaculatory frequency, which often changes with age and may skew semen quality assessments [19]. Moreover, standard semen analysis may not fully capture the nuanced effects of aging on sperm function. For instance, aging has been associated with alterations in the sperm proteome, which may influence proteins critical for motility and fertilization processes [20, 21]. Integrative studies involving proteomics and metabolomics have also shown that older paternal age correlates with changes in protein expression related to oxidative stress and metabolic control [21].

The hypothalamic-pituitary-testicular axis, illustrated in **Figure 1**, demonstrates progressive age-related dysregulation characterized by three key alterations: (1) diminished hypothalamic GnRH pulsatility, (2) attenuated pituitary LH/FSH secretion, and (3) declining testicular Leydig cell responsiveness. This endocrine disruption leads to impaired testosterone production and spermatogenic dysfunction, compounded by testicular microenvironment deterioration and sperm proteome alterations. Clinically, these changes manifest as both reproductive decline (evidenced by reduced fertility rates and poorer assisted reproduction outcomes in older males) and systemic effects, including metabolic disturbances, cardiovascular risks, and

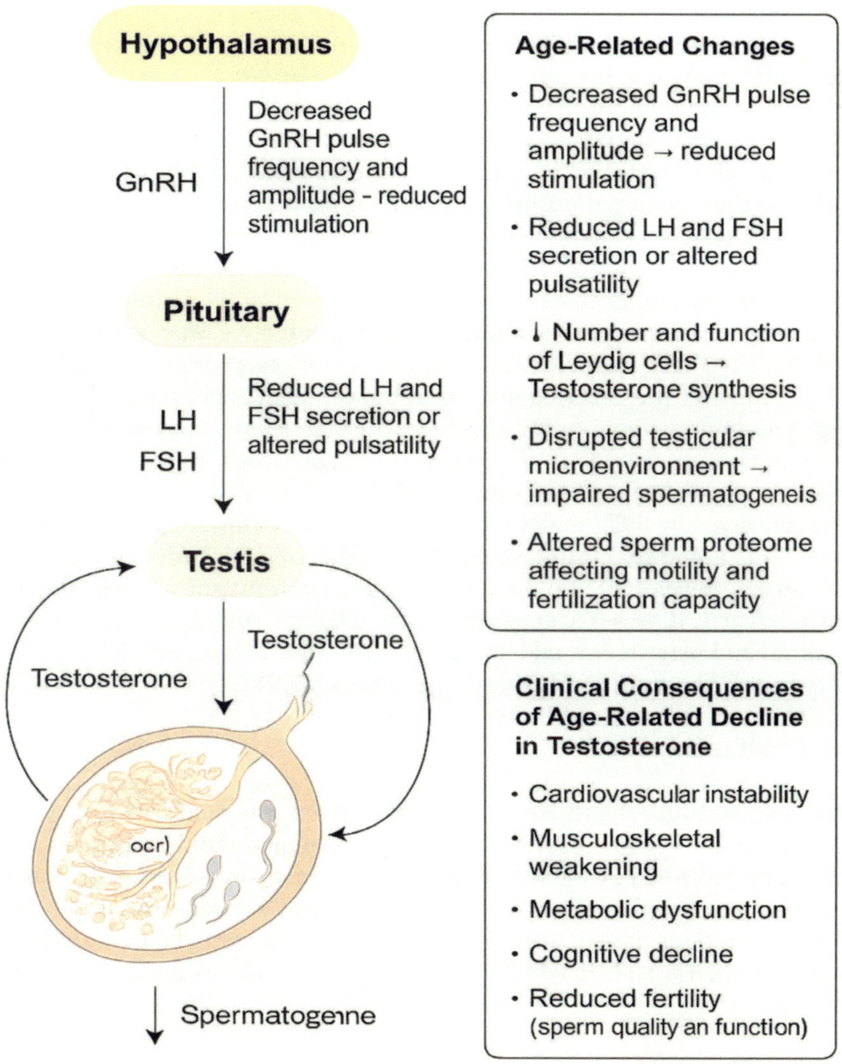

Figure 1.
Age-related decline in the male hypothalamic-pituitary-gonadal (HPG) axis and its clinical consequences.

cognitive changes. This chapter will concentrate specifically on experimental research and meta-analytical findings related to testicular aging, with an emphasis on assessing the impact of diverse therapeutic strategies.

2. Age-related changes in male fertility

Although testicular structure, semen production, and overall reproductive capability are generally maintained in men beyond the age of 50, advancing paternal age has emerged as a notable factor contributing to declining male fertility. Men over the age of 50 demonstrate significantly reduced sperm motility, increased morphological abnormalities, and a higher prevalence of flagellar defects compared to younger men aged 21–25. The decline in fertility potential becomes even more pronounced when both partners are older than 40 years of age [22–24].

Sociodemographic factors, including widespread access to contraception, delayed age at marriage or cohabitation, increased educational attainment, and career prioritization—particularly among women—have collectively contributed to a global trend of postponing parenthood. This postponement is associated with diminished reproductive potential, not only due to the biological impacts of aging on gametes but also due to the accumulation of comorbidities and altered reproductive behaviors that accompany aging. Consequently, the risk of age-related involuntary childlessness rises as the median age at first childbirth continues to increase worldwide [25, 26].

Scientific evidence indicates that increasing paternal age contributes to a greater likelihood of spontaneous genetic alterations in reproductive cells, with particular susceptibility observed in the fibroblast growth factor receptor genes (FGFR2, FGFR3) and the RET proto-oncogene. These molecular changes are etiologically linked to various monogenic conditions following autosomal dominant inheritance patterns, notably craniosynostosis syndromes (Apert, Crouzon, Pfeiffer) and specific endocrine tumor syndromes. Additionally, epidemiological studies demonstrate that offspring conceived by older males face elevated risks of numerical chromosomal aberrations (including sex chromosome aneuploidies and trisomies 13/18) as well as neuropsychiatric developmental disorders ranging from autism spectrum conditions to major psychiatric illnesses. Congenital heart defects involving septal formation abnormalities and persistent fetal circulatory structures also occur with greater frequency in children born to advanced-age fathers [27, 28].

2.1 Sexual malfunction

Sexual dysfunction in all its forms is a major reason why men seek therapy at men's health clinics. The foundation for the logical categorization of human sexual disorders was established by Masters and Johnson's seminal studies of the human sexual response cycle, which showed that both men and women exhibit predictable physiological reactions to sexual stimulation [29]. Consequently, based on the stage of the sexual response cycle in which the aberration occurs, sexual illnesses have been divided into:

1. Disease of hypoactive sexual drives

2. Ejaculation and orgasm disorders

3. Erectile dysfunction

4. Pain disorders

Effective management of male sexual dysfunction requires accurate classification, as each category is associated with distinct underlying causes, diagnostic criteria, and therapeutic strategies. Historically, the classification of sexual disorders was shaped by the *Diagnostic and Statistical Manual of Mental Disorders (DSM)*, which reflected a predominantly psychogenic interpretation of male sexual dysfunction. However, developing clinical insights and the advent of oral phosphodiesterase type 5 (PDE5) inhibitors have shifted the perspective. Erectile dysfunction is now recognized not merely as a psychological issue but often as a marker of broader systemic health problems. As a result, the role of the primary care provider has become increasingly central in the initial evaluation and management of male sexual disorders [30].

2.2 Pathophysiology of age-related reduction of testosterone

The gradual reduction in androgen synthesis observed during male aging stems principally from dysfunction within the neuroendocrine regulatory system connecting the hypothalamus, pituitary gland, and gonads. This multifaceted dysregulation involves both altered hormone metabolism and impaired signaling cascades throughout the endocrine axis. Key pathophysiological changes include: (1) attenuation of GnRH pulse generator activity, (2) loss of synchronous LH secretion patterns from the anterior pituitary, and (3) decreased responsiveness of testicular interstitial cells to gonadotropic stimulation. Additionally, the diurnal variation in androgen secretion—characteristically prominent in younger individuals—shows significant dampening with advancing age, exacerbating the hormonal deficiency state [31, 32]. Clinically, two distinct patterns emerge among aging males with hypogonadism: A minority demonstrate primary gonadal failure with biochemical evidence of elevated gonadotropins, contrasting with low circulating androgens, while the majority present with secondary hypogonadism showing inappropriately normal or low LH levels despite testosterone deficiency. This latter presentation typically reflects systemic metabolic disturbances (particularly adiposity-related endocrine dysfunction) or chronic disease states rather than primary testicular pathology [33].

2.3 Age-related testosterone level

Several breakthrough epidemiological investigations, including the Osteoporotic Fractures in Men Study (MrOS), European Male Aging Study (EMAS), and Framingham Heart Study (FHS), have employed liquid chromatography-tandem mass spectrometry (LC-MS/MS)—considered the reference methodology—to assess circulating androgen levels in male populations. These studies consistently reveal that declining concentrations of both total and unbound testosterone in aging males are predictably correlated with multiple clinical manifestations: diminished sexual desire, compromised erectile capacity, and reduced nocturnal penile tumescence. The same hormonal alterations show significant associations with sarcopenia, self-reported physical limitations, and heightened vulnerability to mobility impairments and accidental falls [34, 35].

The metabolic consequences of androgen deficiency extend to several pathophysiological domains, demonstrating strong correlations with central obesity, impaired glucose homeostasis, and a greater likelihood of developing diabetes mellitus. Further analyses indicate connections between hypogonadism and accelerated biological aging markers (including leukocyte telomere shortening), osteopenia, deterioration of trabecular bone structure, and greater fracture susceptibility. Population-level mortality data suggest that these endocrine changes may influence both cardiovascular outcomes and overall survival. Sex-stratified Mendelian randomization analyses of UK Biobank participants reveal divergent metabolic risk profiles based on genetically influenced androgen levels: while men with a genetic predisposition to lower testosterone show increased type 2 diabetes susceptibility, women with genetically elevated testosterone exhibit comparable metabolic risk. Notably, the same genomic studies identify a potential oncogenic association between androgen-related genetic variants and prostate malignancy in male subjects [35–37].

Overall, the studies conclude that age-related male fertility decline is characterized by reduced sperm motility, increased morphological abnormalities, and flagellar defects after age 50, driven by oxidative stress and mitochondrial dysfunction (**Table 1**) [22–24]. Sociodemographic shifts, such as delayed parenthood, exacerbate these declines, while advanced paternal age elevates risks of de novo mutations (e.g.,*FGFR2/FGFR3*) and neurodevelopmental disorders in offspring

Category	Age-related changes	Physiological mechanisms	References
Semen parameters	↓ Sperm motility, ↑ morphological abnormalities, ↑ flagellar defects after age 50	Oxidative stress accumulation, DNA fragmentation, mitochondrial dysfunction	[22–24]
Genetic risks	↑ De novo mutations (FGFR2, FGFR3, RET), ↑ chromosomal aberrations, ↑ neurodevelopmental disorders in offspring	Epigenetic alterations, reduced DNA repair efficiency in spermatogonial stem cells	[27, 28]
Sexual dysfunction	↓ Libido, erectile dysfunction, orgasmic disorders	↓ Testosterone, endothelial dysfunction, ↑ pro-inflammatory cytokines	[29, 30]
Hormonal decline	↓ Total/free testosterone, dampened diurnal rhythm	HPT axis dysregulation: ↓ GnRH pulsatility, ↓ LH sensitivity, Leydig cell senescence	[31–33]
Metabolic effects	↑ Central obesity, insulin resistance, type 2 diabetes risk	Androgen deficiency → ↑ visceral adiposity → pro-inflammatory state	[35–37]
Musculoskeletal	Sarcopenia, osteopenia, ↑ fracture risk	↓ Testosterone → impaired protein synthesis, ↑ bone resorption	[34, 35]
Systemic health	↑ Cardiovascular risk, ↓ survival	Telomere shortening, chronic inflammation, vascular dysfunction	[34, 35]

↓ = decrease/reduction; ↑ = increase/elevation; GnRH = gonadotropin-releasing hormone; LH = luteinizing hormone; HPT axis = hypothalamic-pituitary-testicular axis; FGFR2 = fibroblast growth factor receptor 2; FGFR3 = fibroblast growth factor receptor 3; RET = REarranged during Transfection proto-oncogene.

Table 1.
Summary of age-related declines in male reproductive and systemic health, including key physiological mechanisms.

due to epigenetic and DNA repair deficits (**Table 1**) [27, 28]. Concurrently, sexual dysfunction (e.g., erectile disorders) and testosterone decline—linked to hypothalamic-pituitary dysregulation—worsen metabolic, musculoskeletal, and cardiovascular health (**Table 1**) [29–37].

3. Intervention to restore age-related testicular complications

Numerous investigations have reported that various interventions can modulate the pathophysiological processes affecting the human testis. Nonetheless, the majority of these studies have focused primarily on the effects of exposure to toxic agents—such as chemotherapeutic drugs (busulfan, cyclophosphamide), environmental contaminants (bisphenol A, cadmium), antiretroviral medications (lopinavir), and physical insults like microwave radiation—or on testicular damage associated with pathological conditions, including diabetes, idiopathic infertility, ischemia-reperfusion injury, and testicular torsion. To date, there remains a paucity of evidence supporting effective therapeutic approaches for the restoration of testicular function in the context of male aging [38].

3.1 Testosterone replacement therapy

Clinical evidence indicates that androgen supplementation therapy offers significant advantages for males with confirmed testosterone deficiency. This intervention demonstrates measurable improvements in skeletal physiology, as evidenced by enhanced bone formation markers and increased mineral density. The treatment modality additionally shows protective effects against urogenital complications, potentially reducing urinary frequency, infection susceptibility, and bladder dysfunction while conferring cardiovascular benefits. Neuropsychiatric manifestations of hypogonadism—including depressive symptoms, emotional dysregulation, and age-related cognitive decline in elderly populations—may show substantial improvement with hormonal normalization [39, 40].

Clinical research investigating androgen replacement in aging males has demonstrated significant therapeutic benefits across multiple physiological systems. A controlled trial involving testicular cancer survivors with Leydig cell impairment (n = 69) revealed that a 12-month intervention with exogenous testosterone yielded measurable improvements in skeletal health parameters compared to placebo, with particular enhancement in bone mineral density metrics and elevated P1NP levels—a specific marker of bone formation activity [41] Complementary demographic research tracking 270 Chinese males across a 50-year age spectrum established a clear inverse relationship between chronological aging and bioavailable androgen concentrations, with free testosterone levels declining progressively after the peak reproductive years [42]. Current therapeutic guidelines endorse testosterone supplementation for confirmed cases of primary hypogonadism, particularly when resulting from intrinsic Leydig cell dysfunction that impairs endogenous steroidogenesis and metabolic regulation. Metabolic studies demonstrate a delayed treatment response pattern, where initial glucose homeostasis parameters remain unchanged during early therapy but show significant improvement in insulin sensitivity after sustained 12-month administration [43]. Cardiovascular monitoring in testosterone-deficient males (mean age 54 years) receiving parenteral testosterone undecanoate revealed clinically relevant blood pressure stabilization within a 4-month treatment window, suggesting potential protective effects against androgen-related hypertension [44]. Geriatric applications show particular promise, with an RCT demonstrating preserved musculoskeletal integrity in octogenarian participants, including maintained femoral bone density and lean body mass composition despite advanced age and obesity [45]. Hematologic benefits extend beyond simple anemia correction, with trial data indicating broader erythropoietic effects that may prevent hematinic deficiencies in at-risk populations [46].

The contemporary understanding of testosterone replacement therapy (TRT) and prostate cancer (PCa) risk presents a complex and often contradictory evidence base. Morgentaler et al. [47] fundamentally challenged the traditional androgen hypothesis by demonstrating that TRT does not increase PCa risk in healthy men, proposing instead the saturation model wherein prostate cancer cell androgen receptors become maximally stimulated at testosterone concentrations of approximately 200 ng/dL. Notably, Wallis et al. [48] conducted a large population-based study (n = 38,570) that revealed significant effect modification by baseline prostate-specific antigen (PSA) levels. While confirming no overall increased PCa risk (HR = 1.01, 95% CI 0.90–1.13), their analysis demonstrated a 47% higher PCa incidence (HR = 1.47, 95% CI 1.04–2.08) among men with baseline PSA >4 ng/mL initiating TRT. This finding directly contradicts the saturation model's universal applicability and suggests either (1) biological stimulation of pre-existing occult cancers by TRT in high-PSA men or (2) detection bias from intensified monitoring. Importantly, Morgentaler's studies systematically excluded this high-PSA population, potentially underestimating TRT-associated risks in clinical practice. Further contradicting the saturation hypothesis, longitudinal data from the Finnish prostate cancer screening cohort by Siltari et al. [49] identified a concerning 76% increase in metastatic PCa risk among former TRT users. This finding implies that TRT cessation, rather than continuous therapy, may paradoxically stimulate cancer progression—a phenomenon unexplained by current receptor saturation models. The temporal pattern of risk elevation (peaking within 2 years post-TRT initiation in Wallis' study and appearing after discontinuation in the Finnish cohort) suggests complex, time-dependent biological interactions not captured by existing paradigms. Clinical guidelines reflect these contradictions. While, according to Khera et al. [50], American Urological Association now permits TRT for men with treated, stable PCa based on the saturation model, it simultaneously acknowledges insufficient evidence for active surveillance patients. This cautious approach contrasts with the FDA's maintained warnings about TRT in all PCa populations, highlighting persistent uncertainty. The guidelines' emphasis on quarterly PSA monitoring for TRT recipients with PCa history indirectly concedes that the saturation model cannot fully assure safety without surveillance.

In conclusion, contemporary evidence suggests that TRT may be safely considered for hypogonadal men with stable, treated prostate cancer, as it demonstrates no increased PCa risk in most cases. However, caution remains for men with elevated PSA (>4 ng/mL) (Wallis) and for former TRT users, highlighting the importance of careful patient selection, PSA monitoring, and shared decision-making (AUA 2022 guidelines). These findings represent a paradigm shift in TRT management, but further research is needed to clarify long-term outcomes.

3.1.1 Long-term effects and safety considerations of testosterone replacement therapy

3.1.1.1 Clinical applications and safety considerations

The administration of exogenous testosterone represents a well-established therapeutic approach for males with confirmed hypogonadism—a clinical condition marked by suboptimal endogenous testosterone production. This intervention demonstrates efficacy in ameliorating characteristic manifestations of androgen deficiency, including persistent fatigue, diminished sexual desire, and progressive loss of lean muscle mass. However, clinicians must carefully evaluate each patient's medical history and current health status before initiating treatment, weighing potential benefits against possible adverse effects, particularly in the context of extended therapeutic regimens. A critical consideration in testosterone supplementation is its potential to worsen existing sleep-disordered breathing, necessitating vigilant monitoring throughout treatment. Effective management requires sustained collaboration between healthcare providers and patients to ensure optimal outcomes. A comprehensive meta-analysis encompassing 51 clinical investigations revealed several significant hematologic alterations associated with androgen therapy:

Erythrocytic effects: Elevated hemoglobin concentrations (mean increase: 0.80 g/dL; 95% CI 0.45–1.14) and hematocrit levels (mean increase: 3.18%; 95% CI 1.35–5.01)

Lipid metabolism: Modest reduction in high-density lipoprotein cholesterol (mean decrease: 0.49 mg/dL; 95% CI −0.85 to −0.13)

Notably, the analysis found no statistically significant association between testosterone replacement and all-cause mortality, prostate-related clinical outcomes, or major cardiovascular events. Contemporary research consistently supports the oncological safety of properly administered androgen therapy in appropriately screened individuals. Multiple study designs—including randomized controlled trials and large-scale epidemiological investigations—demonstrate comparable outcomes between treated and untreated males regarding:

- Prostate gland volume measurements,
- Longitudinal prostate-specific antigen trajectories,
- Incidence rates of benign prostatic hyperplasia progression,
- Development of prostate malignancies.
- These findings collectively suggest that, when implemented with appropriate patient selection and monitoring protocols, testosterone replacement does not appear to increase prostate cancer risk in men without pre-existing prostatic pathology [51].

3.1.1.2 Monitoring protocol

Following the initiation of testosterone supplementation, systematic surveillance is critical to optimize therapeutic outcomes while minimizing risks. The recommended monitoring protocol includes:

3.1.1.2.1 Prostate health assessment

- Digital rectal examination (DRE) and prostate-specific antigen (PSA) testing at 3 and 6 months post-initiation, followed by annual evaluations in patients without prior malignancy,
- More frequent monitoring may be warranted in high-risk populations.

- Comprehensive Laboratory Surveillance
- Hematologic parameters: Hemoglobin and hematocrit levels to assess for erythrocytosis,
- Metabolic profile: Lipid panel (total cholesterol, LDL, HDL, triglycerides) and liver function tests,
- Hormonal evaluation: Testosterone levels (though clinical symptom improvement remains the primary efficacy indicator).
- Special considerations in prostate cancer survivors
- Patients with a history of treated prostate cancer may be candidates for testosterone therapy only after demonstrating:
- No biochemical or clinical evidence of residual disease,
- Stable PSA levels over an appropriate surveillance period,
- Thorough discussion of potential risks and benefits [52].

3.1.1.3 Cardiovascular risk assessment

Current evidence does not substantiate an increased cardiovascular risk with testosterone replacement therapy. Emerging data suggest potential cardioprotective effects, though further investigation is needed to elucidate these relationships [53]. However, before starting a TRT plan, which should be customized based on the patient's unique medical history and concerns, the doctor should completely go over all the advantages and hazards with the patient.

3.2 Corticosteroids hormonal therapy

Low-dose corticosteroids have garnered attention due to their immunomodulatory effects, particularly in the context of idiopathic male infertility. Prednisolone, in particular, has demonstrated the capacity to suppress persistent inflammatory cell infiltration—a histopathological feature frequently observed in testicular biopsies of infertile males. This localized inflammation is often associated with the development of anti-sperm antibodies (ASA), which can compromise sperm function by impairing motility, disrupting zona pellucida binding, or hindering oocyte penetration, ultimately reducing the chances of successful fertilization [54].

Corticosteroids are proposed to enhance male fertility primarily through modulation of the immune system and attenuation of inflammatory responses. By downregulating immune-mediated damage, they may reduce factors that negatively affect sperm function and embryo implantation. For instance, prednisolone has been reported to improve in vitro fertilization (IVF) outcomes and fertility rates in men with anti-sperm antibodies (ASA), suggesting a potential role in mitigating immunologic barriers to fertilization. Additionally, corticosteroids may help resolve chronic inflammation in the male reproductive tract, which is often exacerbated by autoimmune conditions and contributes to impaired spermatogenesis and testicular dysfunction [55]. Previous evidence suggests that, in the absence of ASA, corticosteroids may not significantly improve the reproductive health of men. The chronic corticosteroid treatment has resulted in adverse side effects, such as hormonal imbalances, including low testosterone levels [56, 57].

Although they may have short-term advantages, the possibility of adverse consequences, including immunosuppression, should be carefully considered [58]. It is crucial to weigh the possible advantages and disadvantages of corticosteroid medications, especially because of the other options for treating male infertility, such as ART [58, 59]. In conclusion, further studies are needed to assess the efficacy of low-dose corticosteroids, even if they may provide some therapeutic benefits in the treatment of idiopathic male infertility.

3.3 Antioxidant and anti-inflammatory therapies

3.3.1 Anti-inflammatory therapeutics

Emerging preclinical research has investigated the therapeutic potential of NSAIDs in mitigating age-related testicular dysfunction through various experimental approaches. In vitro studies utilizing aged Leydig cell cultures demonstrate that selective COX-2 inhibition with compounds like NS398 can restore steroidogenic capacity by suppressing pro-inflammatory prostaglandin pathways, leading to enhanced testosterone biosynthesis [60]. Complementary in vivo investigations in aging rodent models reveal that pharmacological COX-2 blockade with specific inhibitors (e.g., DFU) not only elevates serum testosterone levels but also upregulates key steroidogenic proteins, such as StAR [60]. Mechanistic studies have identified $PGF2\alpha$ as a negative regulator of hCG-stimulated androgen production in hamster Leydig cells, while elevated COX-2 expression appears to be a consistent feature of both aged testicular tissue and senescent steroidogenic cells. While numerous NSAIDs (ibuprofen, aspirin, indomethacin, and paracetamol) have been evaluated for their effects on testicular function in younger populations, significant research gaps persist regarding their specific impacts on age-related gonadal decline, warranting further investigation [60–64].

3.3.2 Antioxidant therapeutics

3.3.2.1 Role of oral antioxidants in male reproductive health

Numerous studies have investigated the effects of common oral antioxidants—such as carnitine, vitamins D, C, and E, along with zinc, selenium, and folate—on sperm quality parameters, including motility, morphology, and concentration. While most research has focused on infertility in younger males, fewer studies have explored the therapeutic potential of these antioxidants in aging animal models [65].

3.3.2.1.1 Vitamin D_3 and testicular aging

Vitamin D_3 supplementation has shown promise in counteracting male reproductive aging. In a D-galactose-induced aging rat model, elderly rats received subcutaneous vitamin D_3 at doses ranging from 40 to 400 IU/kg twice weekly for 6 weeks [66]. This intervention aimed to evaluate its protective effects against testicular aging, which is associated with:

- Reduced cellular proliferation,
- Increased apoptosis,
- Elevated oxidative stress,
- Higher levels of advanced glycation end-products (AGEs) in serum and testicular tissue,
- Upregulation of the AGE receptor (AGER).
- Treatment with vitamin D_3 (typically at 100–500 IU/kg/day in related studies) demonstrated significant benefits, including:
- Enhanced testicular cell proliferation,
- Reduced apoptosis,
- Improved antioxidant defenses,
- Decreased oxidative damage.

Additionally, vitamin D_3 suppressed AGER expression while increasing vitamin D receptor (VDR) levels in the testes. Although AGEs remained elevated in aged animals, circulating vitamin D_3 levels were notably reduced. These findings suggest that vitamin D_3 may delay testicular aging by regulating cellular turnover, oxidative stress, and AGE-related signaling pathways [66].

3.3.2.1.2 Impact on testicular function and spermatogenesis

In the same D-galactose-induced aging model (typically administered 100–150 mg/kg/day), vitamin D_3 supplementation (100–500 IU/kg/day) significantly improved:

- Testicular histology,
- Serum testosterone levels,
- Sperm quality.
- Both in vivo and in vitro studies revealed that vitamin D_3 modulates steroidogenic markers in the testes. Key observations included:
- Increased CYP19A1 (aromatase) expression,
- Reduced androgen receptor (AR) levels in both aged and healthy testes,
- A potential estrogen-mediated mechanism supporting spermatogenesis in aging males.

- Notably, vitamin D_3 did not negatively affect spermatogenesis in healthy rats, indicating its ability to maintain hormonal equilibrium between estrogenic and androgenic activity. This balance may play a crucial role in protecting against age-related testicular decline [67].

3.3.2.2 Melatonin's multifaceted role in testicular function and aging

Melatonin is a potent antioxidant with broad-spectrum protective effects across species. Initially evolved to counteract oxidative stress from atmospheric oxygen fluctuations, it exhibits anti-inflammatory, anti-apoptotic, and anti-cancer properties [68]. As a neurohormone primarily secreted by the pineal gland, melatonin crosses the blood-testis barrier to directly modulate testicular functions [69].

3.3.2.2.1 Melatonin and age-related testicular decline

Studies in Syrian hamsters reveal an age-dependent reduction in testicular melatonin levels. Investigations comparing young (6 weeks), adult (15 weeks), and old (2 years) hamsters demonstrated that aging correlates with:

- Declining steroidogenesis: Reduced expression of steroidogenic markers,

- Increased oxidative stress: Elevated NOX, TBARS, and corticosterone, alongside diminished antioxidant enzyme activity (SOD, CAT, GSH-PX).

Notably, melatonin supplementation (0.5–10 mg/kg/day, intraperitoneal/oral) restored steroidogenic activity and antioxidant capacity in aged testes without altering endogenous melatonin or MT1 receptor levels. This suggests that oxidative stress, rather than melatonin deficiency, drives testicular aging [70].

3.3.2.3 Melatonin's variable effects on age-related physiological changes: Experimental evidence

Several studies have investigated melatonin's impact on aging processes in rodent models, revealing both protective effects and limitations. In aged Wistar rats, daily subcutaneous administration of 10 mg/kg melatonin over 3 weeks demonstrated tissue-specific outcomes. While treatment effectively reduced germ cell apoptosis (as evidenced by decreased TUNEL-positive cells) and enhanced seminiferous tubule morphology, it showed no significant effect on age-associated lipid peroxidation markers [71]. This differential response highlights the context-dependent nature of melatonin's antioxidant properties.

Further examination of melatonin's anti-aging potential was conducted by Akbulut and colleagues using a rat model of gastric aging. Their experimental design compared young (4-month-old) and aged (20-month-old) animals, with treatment groups receiving either PBS or melatonin (10 mg/kg, i.p.) for 21 days. Key findings included:

- Significant reduction in gastric mucosal cell proliferation across all age groups,

- Enhanced telomerase activity in both young and aged animals,

- No improvement in glutathione (GSH) levels despite elevated malondialdehyde (MDA) in aged gastric tissue.

These results suggest that while melatonin may influence cellular aging mechanisms such as telomerase activity, its ability to combat oxidative damage in certain tissues may be limited [72].

Recent mechanistic studies have provided insight into melatonin's protective role against environmental toxicants. Wang et al. [73] demonstrated that melatonin administration (2 mg/kg/day, i.p.) protected against cadmium-induced testicular injury in a mouse model through SIRT3-mediated pathways. Their comprehensive approach included:

- In vivo cadmium exposure (0.8 mg/kg/day for 7 days) with melatonin co-treatment in a rat model,
- Parallel in vitro experiments using TM3 Leydig cells (8.725 μg/ml cadmium ± 11 μg/ml melatonin),
- Genetic manipulation (SIRT3 overexpression and knockdown) to confirm SIRT3's essential role in mediating melatonin's protective effects.

The research established that melatonin's regulation of the autophagy-apoptosis balance is dependent on SIRT3 expression, offering potential therapeutic targets for testicular protection. Light exposure conditions appear to modify melatonin's endocrine effects, as shown in studies of testicular steroidogenesis. When administered to rats maintained under normal light-dark cycles (12:12 LD), melatonin (25 μg/100 g) significantly inhibited 17β-HSD and Δ5-3β-HSD enzyme activities. However, this suppressive effect was absent in animals exposed to constant light, despite unchanged serum testosterone levels [74].

3.3.2.4 Novel insights into photoperiodic regulation of testicular aging

Recent studies reveal contrasting therapeutic outcomes between photoperiodic regulation and antioxidant interventions for testicular aging, with Matzkin et al.'s [61] photoperiod manipulation in Syrian hamsters demonstrating superior efficacy by naturally restoring physiological melatonin levels (2.3 ± 0.4 pg./mg) and achieving comprehensive rejuvenation through 62% IL-1β reduction, 73% M1 macrophage decrease, and 2.1-fold claudin-11 increase, whereas conventional antioxidant approaches such as vitamin D_3 supplementation (100–500 IU/kg) and high-dose melatonin (10 mg/kg) showed limited systemic effects, inconsistent oxidative stress modulation, and tissue-specific responses without circadian integration. While photoperiodic regulation simultaneously addressed circadian, immune, redox, and stem cell aging axes, antioxidants exhibited single-pathway efficacy with variable results—melatonin improved telomerase activity but failed to reduce gastric MDA, and vitamin D_3 enhanced local testicular parameters without normalizing macrophage profiles. These findings suggest physiological light-cycle interventions may offer more holistic anti-aging benefits compared to pharmacological antioxidants, highlighting the need for combined approaches that leverage circadian entrainment while optimizing redox balance for complete testicular rejuvenation.

3.3.2.4.1 Methodological advancements of study (Matzkin et al)

- Utilization of naturally aged specimens (24–28 months) rather than chemically induced models,

- Observation across three complete spermatogenic cycles for comprehensive assessment,

- Development of an ecologically valid photoperiod manipulation protocol.

This work resolves long-standing controversies in reproductive aging research by demonstrating that:

- Melatonin's therapeutic effects require intact photoperiodic regulation,

- Physiological hormone concentrations are sufficient for testicular rejuvenation,

- Previous inconsistencies in pharmacological studies stem from disrupted circadian integration.

The study establishes a novel conceptual framework that unifies four critical aspects of male reproductive aging:

- Photoperiod sensitivity,

- Immune privilege maintenance,

- Redox homeostasis,

- Stem cell niche preservation.

The finding of Matzkin et al.'s study has important clinical implications for treating age-related infertility while providing a methodological paradigm that could be adapted to investigate other circadian-regulated aspects of reproductive physiology. The photoperiod manipulation approach represents a significant advancement over traditional supplementation studies, offering more physiologically relevant insights into hormonal regulation [61].

Vitamin D_3 demonstrates efficacy in enhancing steroidogenesis, reducing oxidative stress, and modulating AGE-related pathways in aging models, suggesting its role in preserving testicular function. Melatonin, while exhibiting broad antioxidant and anti-inflammatory properties, shows context-dependent effects, with notable benefits in restoring steroidogenesis and cellular integrity, but a limited impact on lipid peroxidation in certain tissues. Crucially, photoperiodic regulation of endogenous melatonin proves superior to exogenous supplementation, underscoring the importance of circadian biology in therapeutic strategies. These findings collectively emphasize the need for tailored antioxidant interventions that consider hormonal balance, oxidative stress pathways, and physiological timing to effectively address male reproductive aging. Future research should focus on translational approaches that integrate these insights into clinical practice for age-related infertility.

3.4 Emerging pharmacotherapies for male sexual function

Aging is a complex biological process characterized by a progressive decline in cellular function and an increased susceptibility to age-related diseases. This decline is influenced by multiple factors, including telomere attrition, DNA damage, mitochondrial dysfunction, and cellular senescence. These factors contribute to the development of various age-related complications, which can significantly impact the health and well-being of males.

3.4.1 Phosphodiesterase-5 inhibitor (selective)

PDE5 inhibitors, including tadalafil and sildenafil, serve as first-line pharmacological interventions for erectile dysfunction, demonstrating efficacy in restoring sexual function. Concurrently, male infertility has emerged as a growing public health concern in industrialized societies, where psychological, environmental, and physiological stressors contribute to reproductive challenges. These compounds may offer dual therapeutic benefits by addressing both erectile dysfunction and potential fertility impairments through mechanisms involving vascular and cellular effects in the male reproductive system [74]. Males trying to conceive are increasingly adopting PDE5 inhibitors due to their easy accessibility and the high prevalence of male sexual disorders in couples with fertility issues. The possible effects of PDE5 inhibitors on male fertility and semen parameters have thus been the subject of numerous investigations [75, 76]. A prospective clinical trial (Rago et al. [77]) evaluated vardenafil's impact on 205 infertile men using a three-arm design: a control group ($n = 65$) receiving no treatment, an acute intervention group ($n = 73$) administered a single 10 mg dose, and an extended treatment group ($n = 67$) receiving 10 mg every other day for 15 days. Pre- and post-intervention analyses demonstrated that vardenafil significantly improved both erectile function (measured by IIEF-5 scores) and semen parameters, with acute dosing enhancing sperm motility and extended treatment further increasing sperm concentration. These findings suggest vardenafil may benefit male fertility beyond its primary erectile dysfunction indication, potentially through pleiotropic effects on reproductive physiology.

A 12-week randomized clinical trial evaluated the effects of daily vardenafil (Group A, $n = 25$), sildenafil (Group B, $n = 25$), and L-carnitine (Group C, $n = 25$) administration versus untreated controls (Group D, $n = 22$) in 75 men with oligoasthenospermia. Both PDE5 inhibitor groups demonstrated significant post-treatment increases in serum insulin-like peptide 3 (INSL3) levels ($p < 0.01$), along with improvements in sperm concentration (mean increase of 12.5×10^6/mL), motility (28–32% enhancement), and normal morphology (8–11% increase), suggesting these agents may enhance Leydig cell secretory function and subsequently improve semen parameters, while no comparable effects were observed in the L-carnitine or control groups [78].

A controlled laboratory study evaluated the dose- and time-dependent effects of sildenafil citrate (0.1–4.0 mg/mL) on sperm motility in 85 asthenozoospermic specimens using standardized incubation protocols and computerized motility assessment. The results demonstrated a significant concentration-response relationship ($p < 0.05$), with optimal motility enhancement observed at intermediate concentrations (1.0–2.0 mg/mL) that persisted throughout the 3-hour evaluation period. These findings suggest that phosphodiesterase-5 inhibition may directly improve sperm kinematic parameters through cyclic nucleotide-mediated mechanisms, supporting further investigation of sildenafil's potential role in managing male factor infertility, although clinical applications require additional validation of safety and efficacy in vivo [79].

A prospective randomized double-blind crossover trial examined the acute impacts of two phosphodiesterase-5 inhibitors on semen characteristics in 18 young males with confirmed infertility. Participants received single doses of either sildenafil citrate (50 mg) or tadalafil (20 mg) in randomized sequence, with seminal analysis performed 60–120 minutes post-administration using standardized laboratory protocols. The investigation revealed divergent pharmacological effects: sildenafil administration was associated with a 30% relative improvement in progressive sperm motility (median increase from 28.5% to 37.0%), while tadalafil exposure resulted in a 25% reduction (median decrease to 21.5%) compared to baseline values. These contrasting outcomes suggest drug-specific modulation of sperm kinematic properties, potentially mediated through differential pharmacokinetic profiles or distinct intracellular signaling mechanisms. Although the crossover design and blinding procedures minimized potential bias, the preliminary nature of these findings—particularly the unanticipated negative association with tadalafil—necessitates confirmation through larger-scale clinical trials with extended observation periods to establish clinical relevance and elucidate the underlying biological pathways [80].

A systematic evaluation of nine randomized controlled trials (n = 1248 participants) demonstrated that phosphodiesterase-5 inhibitors (sildenafil, tadalafil, and vardenafil) significantly enhance multiple semen parameters in infertile men, showing a 38–42% improvement in sperm concentration ($p < 0.001$), 25–30% increase in progressive motility ($p < 0.001$), and 15–18% higher rates of morphologically normal sperm ($p = 0.005$), while reducing abnormalities by 20–22% ($p < 0.001$). These consistent findings across multiple agents suggest a class effect supporting their potential therapeutic application for male factor infertility, though further research is needed to optimize clinical protocols [81]. While the precise mechanisms remain under investigation, current evidence suggests PDE5 inhibitors may improve sperm quality through multiple pathways: (1) enhanced testicular perfusion via vasodilation of gonadal vasculature, optimizing the spermatogenic microenvironment; (2) direct modulation of sperm function through cGMP-mediated signaling pathways that regulate motility and capacitation; and (3) potential effects on sperm membrane physiology and mitochondrial function. These proposed mechanisms require further validation through controlled studies to establish optimal dosing regimens, treatment duration, and safety profiles, particularly regarding long-term reproductive outcomes in infertile populations [82].

3.4.2 Phosphodiesterase-5 inhibitors (non-selective)

Pentoxifylline and related methylxanthines function as non-selective phosphodiesterase inhibitors and have been shown to improve sperm motility in vitro, which can enhance fertilization success in assisted reproductive technologies (ART). Their mechanism involves increasing intracellular cyclic adenosine monophosphate (cAMP) levels, thereby stimulating sperm movement. However, systemic administration of these agents may not reproduce the same effects observed in vitro, likely due to dilution and distribution throughout the body, which can lower drug concentrations at the target site and potentially induce off-target effects in other tissues [83].

Consequently, non-selective PDE5i have a limited function as stand-alone therapies for male infertility, even if they could be helpful in some ART regimens, especially in sperm preparation for procedures such as intrauterine insemination (IUI)—a type of assisted reproductive technology (ART) used to treat infertility—or in vitro fertilization (IVF). To better address the underlying causes of infertility, additional study is required to improve their usage in fertility treatments and investigate potential combinations with other medications [82].

3.4.3 Maxi-K channel activator

Large-conductance calcium-activated potassium (BK or Maxi-K) channels, which are expressed in arterial and corporal smooth muscle tissues, represent promising therapeutic targets for the treatment of erectile dysfunction (ED). An earlier study tested PDE5 inhibitors (sildenafil, 1 μM) alongside KCa channel activators (NS1619 for BKCa, 10 μM; NS309 for SKCa/IKCa, 1 μM) in human penile arteries, demonstrating that combining these agents synergistically enhanced vasodilation—particularly in diabetic tissues where PDE5 inhibition alone was impaired. In diabetic animal models, this dual therapy restored erectile responses at similar doses, with sildenafil (1–3 mg/kg) paired with KCa openers (NS1619, 1–3 mg/kg) significantly improving blood flow and erection metrics compared to monotherapy. These findings suggest that low-dose KCa activators (1–10 μM in vitro, 1–3 mg/kg in vivo) can potentiate PDE5 inhibitors, offering a promising strategy for diabetic ED resistant to standard treatments [84]. This study by Kun et al. [85] investigated the effects of NS11021, a novel large-conductance calcium-activated potassium (BK) channel opener, on erectile function in rats. The researchers demonstrated that NS11021 (administered at doses of 0.1–10 μM in vitro and 1–3 mg/kg intravenously in vivo) significantly enhanced erectile responses by increasing the relaxation of corpus cavernosum smooth muscle through BK channel activation. The compound was shown to potentiate both electrical field stimulation-induced and nitric oxide-mediated erectile responses in rat penile tissue, while having minimal effects on systemic blood pressure at erectile-enhancing doses. These findings suggest that BK channel openers like NS11021 could represent a promising new therapeutic approach for erectile dysfunction, particularly for cases involving impaired smooth muscle relaxation, with potential advantages over conventional phosphodiesterase-5 inhibitors in terms of targeting the underlying ion channel mechanisms of penile erection. The study provided important preclinical evidence for developing BK channel modulators as potential treatments for erectile dysfunction. This study by Király et al. [86] investigated the role of large-conductance calcium-activated potassium (BK) channels in mediating vascular relaxation in human penile arteries. The researchers demonstrated that BK channels contribute significantly to both nitric oxide (NO)-dependent and endothelium-derived hyperpolarization (EDH)-type relaxation pathways in these vessels. Using pharmacological inhibitors (iberiotoxin, 100 nM) and activators (NS1619, 10 μM) of BK channels, the study showed that these channels work synergistically with NO signaling to regulate penile blood flow. Importantly, the findings revealed that BK channels maintain their functionality even when NO pathways are impaired, suggesting their potential as alternative therapeutic targets for erectile dysfunction, particularly in cases where conventional NO-based treatments are ineffective. The study provided crucial evidence for the dual involvement of BK channels in both major vasorelaxation mechanisms in human penile vasculature.

Collectively, these studies demonstrate that BK (Maxi-K) channel activators represent a promising therapeutic strategy for erectile dysfunction (ED), particularly in cases resistant to conventional PDE5 inhibitors (e.g., diabetic ED). Key findings include:

1. Synergistic effects: Combining PDE5 inhibitors (sildenafil, 1 μM) with BK channel openers (NS1619/NS11021, 1–10 μM in vitro; 1–3 mg/kg in vivo) enhances vasodilation and erectile function, especially in diabetic models where NO signaling is impaired.

2. Dual mechanisms: BK channels contribute to both NO-dependent and endothelium-derived hyperpolarization (EDH)-mediated relaxation in human penile arteries, maintaining functionality even when NO pathways are compromised.

3. Targeted therapy: BK activators (e.g., NS11021) selectively promote corporal smooth muscle relaxation without significant systemic blood pressure effects, offering a potential advantage over PDE5 inhibitors.

These findings support the development of BK channel-targeted therapies as novel treatments for ED, particularly for patients with vascular complications or poor response to existing drugs. Further clinical studies are needed to validate their efficacy and safety in humans.

3.4.4 Guanylate cyclase activator

Guanylate cyclase (GC) activators hold significant therapeutic promise for male health by directly stimulating cGMP production, offering distinct advantages for treating erectile dysfunction (ED), particularly in cases resistant to conventional PDE5 inhibitors such as sildenafil. By targeting soluble GC (sGC), these compounds (e.g., BAY 60-4552, riociguat) enhance cavernosal smooth muscle relaxation and penile blood flow even when nitric oxide bioavailability is compromised, as commonly occurs in diabetes, hypertension, and aging-related endothelial dysfunction. Preclinical and clinical studies demonstrate that GC activators can synergize with PDE5 inhibitors to restore erectile function in treatment-resistant ED, while also conferring cardiovascular benefits through improved endothelial function and blood pressure regulation. This study by Albersen et al. [87] investigated a novel therapeutic approach for PDE5 inhibitor-resistant erectile dysfunction by examining the combined effects of BAY 60-4552 (a soluble guanylate cyclase stimulator) and vardenafil (a PDE5 inhibitor) on human corpus cavernosum tissue, demonstrating that the two agents act synergistically (at concentrations of 0.1–10 μM and 0.001–1 μM, respectively) to enhance smooth muscle relaxation through complementary mechanisms—with BAY 60-4552 increasing cGMP production and vardenafil preventing its degradation—thereby effectively restoring erectile tissue responsiveness in previously treatment-resistant cases and suggesting a promising dual-target strategy for managing PDE5 inhibitor-refractory erectile dysfunction. This study by Silva et al. [88] demonstrated that chronic administration (4 weeks) of the soluble guanylyl cyclase (sGC) activator BAY 60-2770 (1 mg/kg/day) effectively restored erectile function in obese mice by bypassing impaired nitric oxide signaling and directly stimulating the NO-sGC-cGMP pathway in penile tissue. The treatment specifically improved both neurogenic and endothelium-dependent erectile responses without causing systemic hypotension, highlighting its tissue-selective action. These findings provided important preclinical evidence that sGC activators like BAY 60-2770 could offer a promising therapeutic approach for metabolic syndrome-associated erectile dysfunction, particularly in cases where conventional PDE5 inhibitors fail due to underlying endothelial dysfunction. The study further suggested that prolonged sGC activation might reverse, rather than just temporarily alleviate, the vascular pathology contributing to obesity-related erectile dysfunction.

In conclusion, these compounds demonstrate tissue-selective effects, improving cavernosal relaxation and penile blood flow without causing systemic hypotension, suggesting their potential as next-generation therapies for metabolic and vascular ED, where conventional PDE5 inhibitors often fail. The findings highlight sGC activators' unique ability to address the root vascular pathology in ED rather than just the symptoms, positioning them as particularly valuable for patients with underlying endothelial damage.

3.4.5 Nitric oxide donors

Nitric oxide (NO) serves as the principal mediator of erectile function, primarily released from cavernous nerve terminals and, to a lesser extent, from endothelial cells of penile arteries. The amino acid precursor L-arginine stimulates endothelial NO synthesis through its role as a substrate for nitric oxide synthase. Clinical investigation of a novel combination therapy (8 g L-arginine aspartate plus 200 mg adenosine monophosphate) demonstrated significant therapeutic efficacy in a phase II trial involving 26 patients with erectile dysfunction. Treated subjects exhibited statistically significant improvements in both erection hardness scores (EHS) and International Index of Erectile Function-5 (IIEF-5) questionnaire results compared to placebo controls. The therapeutic formulation showed excellent tolerability, with no reports of serious adverse events during the study period [89]. This randomized clinical trial by El-Wakeel et al. [90] evaluated the efficacy of combining sildenafil citrate (50 mg on-demand) with L-arginine (1000 mg twice daily) versus sildenafil monotherapy (50 mg on-demand) in patients with organic erectile dysfunction. Over 12 weeks, the combination group demonstrated significantly greater improvements in IIEF-5 scores and penile hemodynamics (Doppler ultrasound) compared to sildenafil alone, attributable to their complementary mechanisms: L-arginine enhanced nitric oxide (NO) synthesis by providing substrate for endothelial NO synthase, while sildenafil preserved cGMP via PDE5 inhibition. The selected L-arginine dose (1000 mg BID) was optimized for bioavailability and synergy with sildenafil without compromising tolerability—no severe adverse events were reported in either group. These findings support the therapeutic advantage of dual-pathway targeting (NO production + cGMP preservation) in organic ED, particularly for cases involving endothelial dysfunction, while maintaining the safety profile of standard sildenafil therapy.

The referenced study, conducted by Futura Medical Developments Ltd. and registered on ClinicalTrials.gov (NCT04008732), evaluated the bioavailability of MED2005, a topical glyceryl trinitrate (GTN) gel for erectile dysfunction, at different doses (0.2%, 0.4%, and 0.6% GTN) in comparison to Nitrostat® (0.4 mg sublingual nitroglycerin), a standard treatment for angina. The trial aimed to assess how effectively each dose of MED2005 delivered nitroglycerin into systemic circulation compared to the rapid absorption of Nitrostat. By analyzing pharmacokinetic and pharmacodynamic responses, researchers sought to determine whether the topical gel could provide localized vasodilation (enhancing penile blood flow) at therapeutic doses while minimizing systemic side effects, such as hypotension. This study was crucial in establishing the optimal dose of MED2005 for further clinical development as a potential on-demand treatment for erectile dysfunction, particularly in patients who may not tolerate oral phosphodiesterase-5 (PDE5) inhibitors due to cardiovascular risks. The full trial details, including methodology and outcomes, are available through the U.S. National Library of Medicine's clinical trial registry [91].

This randomized crossover study by Ralph et al. [92] evaluated the efficacy and safety of MED2005, a topical glyceryl trinitrate (GTN) gel administered at doses of 0.2%, 0.4%, and 0.6%, for treating erectile dysfunction (ED). The double-blind, placebo-controlled trial involved men with mild-to-moderate ED who applied either MED2005 (at varying concentrations) or a placebo gel before sexual activity. Results demonstrated dose-dependent improvements, with the 0.4% and 0.6% doses showing significantly better erectile function compared to placebo, including higher success rates for penetration and maintaining erections. While all doses were generally well-tolerated, the most common side effect was mild headaches (attributed to systemic GTN absorption), which increased slightly with higher concentrations. The study suggests that MED2005, particularly at the 0.4% dose, could serve as an effective on-demand treatment alternative for ED patients, offering rapid onset (~5–15 minutes) and potential advantages for those who cannot take oral phosphodiesterase-5 inhibitors [92].

In conclusion, nitric oxide (NO) donors such as L-arginine and glyceryl trinitrate (GTN) play a significant role in the management of erectile dysfunction by enhancing endothelial NO availability and promoting vasodilation. Clinical evidence supports their efficacy, particularly when used in combination therapies or as topical formulations like MED2005, offering rapid onset and favorable safety profiles. These approaches provide promising alternatives or adjuncts to traditional PDE5 inhibitors, especially for patients with endothelial dysfunction or those who are unable to tolerate oral medications.

3.4.6 Dopamine agonists

Infertility and hyperprolactinemia are caused by a pituitary adenoma that secretes prolactin. When pulsatile GnRH production is inhibited by high prolactin levels, it can result in male infertility and hypogonadism. Dopamine agonists were suggested as a therapy for pituitary tumors and infertility. Cabergoline and bromocriptine were used as therapeutics in the past. Nonetheless, it was demonstrated that cabergoline suppresses prolactin production better than bromocriptine and restores prolactin levels to normal in 70% of individuals who are resistant to it [93]. Cabergoline, administered at doses ranging from 0.125 to 1.0 mg twice weekly, is the treatment of choice for hyperprolactinemia due to its superior efficacy in normalizing serum prolactin levels and reducing prolactinoma size. Patients who fail to achieve normoprolactinemia at the highest tolerated dose exhibit less than a 50% reduction in tumor volume, or do not experience restoration of fertility are considered resistant to dopamine agonist therapy. In such cases, therapeutic strategies typically involve dose escalation or transitioning from bromocriptine to cabergoline. However, bromocriptine has not demonstrated significant efficacy compared to placebo in the management of idiopathic oligozoospermia [94]. In conclusion, dopamine agonists such as cabergoline have demonstrated high efficacy in the management of infertility associated with hyperprolactinemia; however, their therapeutic benefit in cases of idiopathic male infertility remains limited. Advancing a comprehensive understanding of the diverse etiologies underlying male infertility is crucial for the development of targeted and effective treatment strategies. Further research is warranted to elucidate the specific roles of dopamine agonists and to explore additional therapeutic approaches in the context of idiopathic infertility [82].

3.4.7 Kallikrein

Research has identified bradykinin and kallidin as biologically active peptides that participate in localized inflammatory responses through kallikrein-mediated cleavage of kininogen substrates. In reproductive biology, this enzymatic system appears to influence sperm movement characteristics, as evidenced by laboratory investigations. Clinical research employing rigorous methodology has substantiated these findings—a randomized, double-blind crossover study administering 600 kallikrein units daily over 2 months reported measurable enhancements in semen quality metrics, accompanied by a notable increase in conception probability from a baseline of 18–38% among participants [95]. Our research team has previously documented beneficial effects of kallikrein administration on male fertility parameters [96]. Of particular concern are reports indicating exacerbation of inflammatory pathologies in the prostate and epididymal tissues following treatment [97]. These findings collectively underscore the dual nature of kallikrein intervention—while offering promising fertility enhancement for select patients, the therapy carries measurable clinical risks. This dichotomy necessitates the development of personalized treatment protocols that carefully weigh potential benefits against possible complications. Future investigations should prioritize establishing evidence-based guidelines for patient selection, dosage optimization, and safety monitoring to facilitate responsible clinical application of this therapeutic approach [82].

3.4.8 Indomethacin

Research indicates that prostaglandins exert inhibitory effects on testicular function, suppressing both steroid hormone production and spermatogenesis while impairing sperm motility in laboratory settings. These observations suggest prostaglandins may serve as physiological regulators that negatively modulate male reproductive capacity, implying that their pharmacological inhibition could potentially enhance fertility outcomes. Clinical investigations support this hypothesis—a well-designed study by Barkay and colleagues demonstrated that therapeutic administration of either indomethacin (75 mg daily) or ketoprofen significantly elevated circulating levels of FSH, LH, and testosterone. This hormonal modulation was associated with measurable improvements in semen quality parameters, including enhanced sperm motility and concentration, ultimately achieving a 35% pregnancy rate among treated subjects [98]. While these findings position prostaglandin inhibition as a promising intervention for certain forms of male infertility, particularly in cases characterized by elevated prostaglandin activity, several important considerations remain. The current evidence base necessitates further rigorous investigation to: (1) identify optimal candidate selection criteria, (2) develop targeted treatment protocols, and (3) establish comprehensive risk-benefit profiles for specific patient populations [82]. Future research directions should focus on elucidating the precise mechanisms underlying these therapeutic effects while developing clinically relevant biomarkers to guide treatment decisions.

3.4.9 Alpha-blockers

Preclinical investigations using rodent models have demonstrated that pharmacological blockade of alpha-adrenergic receptors can stimulate testicular spermatogenesis and elevate sperm counts in the epididymis, suggesting that these receptors may regulate male reproductive physiology [99]. Mechanistic studies reveal that alpha-adrenergic antagonists modulate sperm transport dynamics within both the testicular and epididymal compartments, potentially influencing male fertility parameters [100]. Clinical translation of these findings has identified terazosin, a selective alpha-1 blocker, as a candidate treatment for idiopathic oligozoospermia, with human trials reporting measurable improvements in seminal parameters, particularly in sperm concentration [101]. While these preliminary results indicate therapeutic promise for alpha-blockers in specific male infertility cases, the current evidence base remains insufficient to establish definitive clinical guidelines. Further research is required to fully characterize the risk-benefit profile of these agents and determine their precise role in fertility management protocols [82].

Emerging pharmacotherapies for male sexual function and infertility target diverse physiological pathways, reflecting the multifactorial nature of these conditions. Phosphodiesterase-5 inhibitors (both selective and non-selective) have demonstrated consistent efficacy in improving erectile function and, in some cases, enhancing semen parameters such as sperm motility, concentration, and morphologies. New therapeutic strategies, such as Maxi-K channel activators and soluble guanylate cyclase stimulators, offer promising alternatives or adjuncts, particularly for individuals with treatment-resistant or vascular-related erectile dysfunction. Nitric oxide donors, either as dietary supplements or topical agents, provide additional benefits through enhanced endothelial function and a rapid onset of action. Dopamine agonists like cabergoline remain the gold standard for hyperprolactinemia-associated infertility but show limited benefit in idiopathic cases. Other agents, such as kallikrein, indomethacin, and alpha-blockers, have shown variable outcomes and highlight the importance of patient-specific factors in therapeutic decision-making. Overall, while several pharmacologic agents show potential in improving male sexual function and fertility, further high-quality clinical studies are essential to establish optimal treatment regimens, clarify mechanisms of action, and ensure long-term safety and efficacy.

Overall, the studies conclude that emerging pharmacotherapies for male sexual dysfunction and infertility, as summarized in **Table 2**, target diverse physiological pathways, with selective PDE5 inhibitors (e.g., sildenafil, vardenafil) demonstrating dual benefits for erectile function and semen parameters, including improved sperm motility, concentration, and morphologies, though drug-specific variability exists, as tadalafil unexpectedly reduced motility in one study. Novel approaches like Maxi-K channel activators (e.g., NS1619, 1–3 mg/kg) and guanylate cyclase stimulators (e.g., BAY 60-2770, 1 mg/kg/day) show promise for PDE5 inhibitor-resistant cases, particularly in diabetic ED, by synergizing with existing therapies or bypassing impaired NO signaling, while nitric oxide donors like topical MED2005 (0.4% GTN gel) and oral L-arginine (1000 mg BID) offer rapid-onset alternatives for endothelial dysfunction. In contrast, dopamine agonists (e.g., cabergoline, 0.125–1.0 mg twice weekly) are effective only for hyperprolactinemia-associated infertility, and kallikrein (600 kU/day) improves pregnancy rates but carries inflammatory risks, whereas indomethacin (75 mg/day) and alpha-blockers like terazosin show variable efficacy in idiopathic cases, underscoring the need for personalized, mechanism-driven therapies and further clinical validation, as comprehensively outlined in **Table 2**.

3.5 Emerging combination therapies in male infertility management

Contemporary approaches to male infertility treatment increasingly focus on multimodal therapeutic strategies that integrate hormonal modulation with

Therapy type	Mechanism of action	Route and doses	Main findings	References
PDE5 inhibitors (selective)	Inhibits PDE5 → ↑ cGMP → smooth muscle relaxation → improved penile blood flow.	• Vardenafil: 10 mg single dose • Sildenafil: 50 mg single dose • Tadalafil: 20 mg single dose	• Improved sperm motility, concentration, and morphology. • Increased serum INSL3 (Leydig cell function). • Sildenafil enhanced sperm motility in vitro; tadalafil reduced it.	[77, 79–81]
PDE5 inhibitors (non-selective)	Non-specific PDE inhibition → ↑ cAMP → improved sperm motility.	• Pentoxifylline: In vitro use in ART (dose not specified)	• Limited systemic efficacy; useful in ART for sperm preparation. • No standalone benefit for male infertility.	[82, 83]
Maxi-K channel activators	Opens BK channels → smooth muscle hyperpolarization → vasodilation.	• NS1619/NS11021: 1–10 μM (in vitro), 1–3 mg/kg (in vivo)	• Synergistic with PDE5 inhibitors in diabetic ED. • Effective in NO-deficient conditions. • Minimal systemic hypotension.	[84–86]
Guanylate cyclase activators	Directly stimulates sGC → ↑ cGMP → vasodilation.	• BAY 60-4552/BAY 60-2770: 0.1–10 μM (in vitro), 1 mg/kg/day (in vivo)	• Restored erectile function in obese/PDE5-resistant ED. • Tissue-selective (no systemic hypotension).	[87, 88]
Nitric oxide donors	• L-arginine: ↑ NO synthesis. • GTN (MED2005): Releases NO → vasodilation.	• L-arginine: 1000 mg BID + sildenafil 50 mg • MED2005: 0.2%, 0.4%, 0.6% topical gel.	• L-arginine + sildenafil improved IIEF-5 scores. • MED2005 (0.4% dose) showed rapid onset (~5–15 min) and efficacy in mild–moderate ED.	[89–92]
Dopamine agonists	Suppresses prolactin → restores GnRH pulsatility → improves hypogonadism/ infertility.	• Cabergoline: 0.125–1.0 mg twice weekly.	• Effective for hyperprolactinemia-induced infertility. • No benefit in idiopathic oligozoospermia.	[93, 94]
Kallikrein	↑ Kinins → modulates sperm motility.	• 600 kU/day for 60 days.	• Improved sperm parameters/pregnancy rates (18% → 38%). • Risk of worsening inflammation.	[95–97]

DOI: http://dx.doi.org/10.5772/intechopen.1012430

Therapy type	Mechanism of action	Route and doses	Main findings	References
Indomethacin	Inhibits prostaglandins → ↑ FSH/LH/testosterone → improved spermatogenesis.	• 75 mg/day	• Increased sperm motility/concentration; 35% pregnancy rate. • Limited clinical evidence.	[98]
Alpha-blockers	Blocks α-adrenergic receptors → ↑ sperm concentration.	• Terazosin: Dose not specified	• Beneficial in idiopathic oligozoospermia. • Mechanism unclear; requires further study.	[99–101]

↓ = decrease/reduction ↑ = increase/elevation; PDE5 = phosphodiesterase type 5 (enzyme inhibition improves erectile function); cGMP = cyclic guanosine monophosphate (secondary messenger in vasodilation); cAMP = cyclic adenosine monophosphate (secondary messenger in sperm motility); ART = assisted reproductive technology (in vitro sperm preparation); BK channels = big potassium channels (smooth muscle relaxation); NO = nitric oxide (vasodilation and erectile function); sGC = soluble guanylate cyclase (enzyme activated by NO); GTN = glyceryl trinitrate (topical NO donor); IIEF-5 = International Index of Erectile Function 5-item (ED severity assessment); GnRH = gonadotropin-releasing hormone (regulates reproductive hormones); FSH = follicle-stimulating hormone (spermatogenesis regulation); LH = luteinizing hormone (testosterone production); INSL3 = insulin-like peptide 3 (Leydig cell biomarker); ED = erectile dysfunction (primary condition treated); BID = Bis in die (twice daily, dosing frequency).

Table 2.
Emerging pharmacotherapies for male sexual dysfunction: Comparative mechanisms of action, administration routes, dosing regimens, and clinical outcomes.

complementary pharmacological agents. Current clinical evidence suggests that co-administration of conventional hormonal treatments with antioxidant supplements yields superior outcomes in idiopathic cases compared to monotherapy approaches. Particularly noteworthy are treatment regimens combining tamoxifen citrate with bioactive plant-derived compounds, such as *Ecklonia bicyclis* and *Tribulus terrestris*. These synergistic combinations have demonstrated clinically meaningful improvements across multiple semen parameters, including substantial enhancements in both sperm density and kinetic characteristics. Importantly, such combined protocols show greater efficacy in achieving successful conception outcomes relative to isolated tamoxifen administration, as documented in recent clinical investigations [102].

3.5.1 Antioxidant combination vs. hormonal combination therapies

Current therapeutic approaches for male infertility increasingly explore synergistic combinations of pharmacological agents. Several randomized controlled trials have examined protocols combining antioxidants (vitamin E, L-carnitine) with anti-estrogen medications (clomiphene), demonstrating variable effects on semen parameters and conception rates [103, 104]. While some commercial antioxidant formulations containing N-acetylcysteine and multivitamin complexes show modest improvements in select sperm quality markers, these changes frequently fail to correlate with increased natural conception probabilities [105]. Similarly, supplementation regimens incorporating zinc, selenium, and various vitamins yield inconsistent results, with some studies reporting enhanced sperm motility and concentration while others show limited clinical impact [106]. The hormonal combination of tamoxifen citrate with testosterone undecanoate has emerged as a more promising intervention for idiopathic oligozoospermia. A placebo-controlled trial involving 212 affected men revealed that 6 months of combined therapy significantly improved total sperm count, motility, and morphology compared to placebo. Most notably, the treatment group achieved a 3.3-fold higher spontaneous pregnancy rate (33.9% vs. 10.3%), suggesting genuine therapeutic potential for this specific combination [107]. Current therapeutic strategies for male infertility focus on optimizing endogenous hormone regulation through targeted pharmacological interventions. Selective estrogen receptor modulators (SERMs), including clomiphene citrate (25–50 mg administered either daily or on alternate days) and tamoxifen citrate (10–20 mg twice daily), represent first-line options that enhance pituitary gonadotropin secretion to promote testicular testosterone synthesis and spermatogenic function. For patients exhibiting hormonal imbalances characterized by elevated estradiol or suboptimal testosterone-to-estradiol ratios, aromatase inhibitors such as anastrozole (1 mg daily) or letrozole (2.5 mg daily) offer an alternative mechanism to restore physiological androgen levels [108, 109]. Importantly, exogenous testosterone administration remains contraindicated due to its well-documented suppression of the hypothalamic-pituitary-gonadal axis, which reduces intratesticular testosterone concentrations and impairs sperm production. Despite this evidence, clinical practice surveys reveal persistent off-label testosterone use among both general urologists and fertility specialists, underscoring the need for improved therapeutic guidelines [110]. The current evidence suggests that while various antioxidant and hormonal combinations may improve semen parameters, only specific regimens (particularly tamoxifen-testosterone undecanoate) demonstrate consistent pregnancy outcome benefits. Optimal treatment strategies should prioritize agents that stimulate rather than suppress endogenous hormone production, with careful consideration of individual patient characteristics in idiopathic male infertility cases.

3.5.2 Emerging combinations

Recent advances in reproductive medicine have led to the development of novel combination therapies targeting specific etiologies of male factor infertility. Clinical studies demonstrate that co-administration of anastrozole with clomiphene citrate yields superior outcomes compared to anastrozole monotherapy, with statistically significant improvements in post-treatment sperm concentration parameters [111]. Similarly, promising results have emerged from protocols combining human chorionic gonadotropin (hCG) with letrozole in obese patients with idiopathic infertility, showing measurable enhancements across multiple semen parameters, including sperm morphology, concentration, and progressive motility [112]. These combination approaches offer several potential advantages:

1. Synergistic mechanisms targeting multiple pathways,
2. Improved efficacy compared to single-agent regimens,
3. Potential for dose reduction of individual components,
4. Better tolerance profiles.

However, current evidence presents notable limitations:

- Variability in treatment response among patient subgroups,
- Lack of standardized dosing protocols,
- Insufficient data on long-term outcomes,
- Limited cost-effectiveness analyses.

Future research directions should prioritize:

1. Multicenter randomized controlled trials with adequate power,
2. Standardization of treatment protocols,
3. Development of predictive biomarkers,
4. Comprehensive safety assessments,
5. Patient stratification based on clinical characteristics.

These combination strategies represent a paradigm shift in male infertility treatment, moving beyond empirical monotherapy toward personalized, pathophysiology-based approaches. While preliminary results are encouraging, rigorous clinical validation remains essential before their widespread implementation [82].

3.6 Lifestyle interventions

Lifestyle interventions and molecular therapies represent distinct but increasingly intertwined approaches to health and disease management. Lifestyle interventions focus on modifying daily habits and behaviors to improve overall health and well-being. These interventions typically encompass dietary changes, increased physical activity, stress management techniques, and avoidance of harmful behaviors, such as smoking and excessive alcohol consumption. Molecular therapies, on the other hand, target specific biological pathways or molecules involved in disease processes. These therapies often involve drugs, gene therapies, or other interventions designed to correct or modulate specific molecular mechanisms [113]. Age-related physiological changes manifest across multiple organ systems, with endocrine alterations presenting particular clinical significance. Research has established a correlation between declining androgen levels and elevated depressive symptomology in aging male populations [114]. Epidemiological evidence further reveals that hypovitaminosis D represents an independent risk factor for late-onset mood disorders in this demographic. The interdependent relationship between vitamin D status and testosterone bioavailability suggests a potential mechanistic link, in which vitamin D sufficiency may confer psychological benefits through endocrine modulation. These findings support clinical recommendations for vitamin D supplementation or controlled sunlight exposure as preventive strategies against affective disorders in middle-aged and elderly men [115].

Participants showed contradictory views about their aging bodies in a research examining how males between the ages of 65 and 83 viewed changes in appearance, physical function, and health as they aged. According to the findings, older men expressed a variety of concerns about specific changes in their bodies as they aged, highlighting the need to address these changes while maintaining a realistic awareness of the complex emotions associated with aging. Participants showed a dedication to exercise and a nutritious diet in spite of their reservations. Therefore, raising awareness and educating males about psychological adaptability during the aging process is crucial [116].

Effective adaptation to the aging process requires men to maintain active engagement in both social interactions and physical pursuits. A comprehensive understanding of how males navigate physiological transformations within their interpersonal relationships is essential for developing appropriate support systems [117]. Central to this understanding is the assessment of hormonal factors, particularly androgen levels, which necessitates multimodal evaluation approaches to capture the complex interplay of biological and psychosocial elements [118]. Body image perception demonstrates gender-specific patterns, with body mass index (BMI) serving as the primary metric for physical appearance satisfaction across both sexes. However, research reveals that men tend to evaluate their attractiveness more strongly through functional physical capabilities rather than purely esthetic considerations [119]. The psychological impact of aging presents significant quality-of-life implications, particularly when negative self-perceptions develop. Targeted mental health interventions should therefore be prioritized for aging males experiencing psychological distress, with a focus on enhancing coping mechanisms and promoting positive aging perspective [120].

The gradual loss of muscle mass, beginning as early as age 30 and accelerating after 50, significantly impacts daily function in aging men [121]. Research highlights the protective role of physical activity, with active individuals showing a lower risk of age-related symptoms (adjusted OR = 0.8, 95% CI: 0.6–1.0) compared to sedentary peers (adjusted OR = 0.7, 95% CI: 0.6–0.9), alongside improvements in somatic ($p < 0.01$) and sexual health ($p = 0.04$) on the Aging Males' Symptoms (AMS) scale [122]. Additionally, aerobic exercise preserves vascular function in older men by reducing oxidative stress and maintaining nitric oxide bioavailability, supporting endothelial health [123].

For aging men, a combination of regular exercise and targeted nutritional supplementation helps maintain reproductive function. Engaging in 150 minutes of moderate aerobic activity (e.g., brisk walking) weekly, in addition to 2–3 days of resistance training, improves testosterone levels, erectile function, and metabolic health [124, 125]. Mind-body practices such as yoga or tai chi (twice weekly) further support hormonal balance by reducing stress. Nutritionally, vitamin D3 (1000–2000 IU/day) enhances testosterone and semen quality, particularly in deficient individuals, while a combination of antioxidants—including zinc (15–30 mg), vitamin E (200–400 IU), vitamin C (500–1000 mg), CoQ10 (100–300 mg), omega-3 s (1000–2000 mg EPA + DHA), and B vitamins (400 mcg folate +2.4 mcg B12)—supports testicular function and reduces oxidative stress [126–131].

4. Conclusion

Testicular aging involves progressive structural and functional decline, leading to reduced testosterone production and significant clinical consequences, including sexual dysfunction, metabolic disturbances, bone density loss, mood alterations, and cognitive changes, while advanced paternal age correlates with decreased fertility and increased risks of genetic mutations (particularly in FGFR2, FGFR3, and RET genes), chromosomal abnormalities, and developmental disorders in offspring. The underlying pathophysiology reflects hypothalamic-pituitary-testicular axis dysregulation, diminished steroidogenic capacity, and impaired feedback mechanisms, often coinciding with metabolic complications, such as central adiposity and insulin resistance. Current management approaches include testosterone replacement therapy for hypogonadism, which demonstrates benefits for bone, urological, and cardiovascular health, alongside investigational agents targeting various pathways, such as phosphodiesterase inhibitors, dopaminergic compounds, and anti-inflammatory medications. Emerging evidence supports combined antioxidant-hormonal regimens as promising interventions for preserving spermatogenesis, though optimal treatment requires personalized strategies based on clinical evidence and individual patient factors, emphasizing the need for continued research to refine therapeutic approaches for aging male reproductive health.

Abbreviations

AMPK	AMP-activated protein kinase
AR	androgen receptor
ART	assisted reproductive technology
ASD	autism spectrum disorder
BAX	Bcl-2 associated X protein
BCL-2	B-cell lymphoma 2
BMI	body mass index

CAT	catalase
CoQ10	coenzyme Q10
DHA	docosahexaenoic acid
DHEA	dehydroepiandrosterone
DNA	deoxyribonucleic acid
DSM	diagnostic and statistical manual of mental disorders
ED	erectile dysfunction
ELISA	enzyme-linked immunosorbent assay
EMAS	European male aging study
EPA	eicosapentaenoic acid
FGFR2	fibroblast growth factor receptor 2
FGFR3	fibroblast growth factor receptor 3
FHS	framingham Heart Study
FSH	follicle-stimulating hormone
GnRH	gonadotropin-releasing hormone
GPx	glutathione peroxidase
H&E	hematoxylin and eosin (staining)
HPG	hypothalamic-pituitary-gonadal (axis)
HPT	hypothalamic-pituitary-testicular (axis)
ICSI	intracytoplasmic sperm injection
IUI	intrauterine insemination
IVF	in vitro fertilization
LC–MS/MS	liquid chromatography-tandem mass spectrometry
LD	long day (photoperiod)
LH	luteinizing hormone
MDA	malondialdehyde
MrOS	osteoporotic fractures in men study
mTOR	mechanistic target of rapamycin
NAC	N-acetylcysteine
NO	nitric oxide
OS	oxidative stress
PDE5	phosphodiesterase type 5
RETS	rearranged during transfection proto-oncogene
ROS	reactive oxygen species
SD	short day (photoperiod)
SDH	succinate dehydrogenase
SOD	superoxide dismutase
T2DM	type 2 diabetes mellitus
TRT	testosterone replacement therapy
TUNEL	terminal deoxynucleotidyl transferase dUTP nick-end labeling

Author details

Shabnoor Iqbal[1*] and Usman Mir Khan[2]

1 AMITD Department of Pharmacology, School of Clinical Medicine, Faculty of Health Sciences, University of the Free State, Bloemfontein, South Africa

2 National Institute of Food Science and Technology, University of Agriculture, Faisalabad, Pakistan

*Address all correspondence to: shabnooriqbal@gcuf.edu.pk; iqbal.s@ufs.ac.za

References

[1] Li L, Papadopoulos V. Advances in stem cell research for the treatment of primary hypogonadism. Nature Reviews Urology. 2021;**18**(8):487-507. DOI: 10.1038/s41585-021-00480-2

[2] Cui L, Nie X, Guo Y, Ren P, Guo Y, Wang X, et al. Single-cell transcriptomic atlas of the human testis across the reproductive lifespan. Nature Aging. 2025;**5**(4):658-674. DOI: 10.1038/s43587-025-00824-2

[3] Anawalt BD, Matsumoto AM. Aging and androgens: Physiology and clinical implications. Reviews in Endocrine and Metabolic Disorders. 2022;**23**(6):1123-1137. DOI: 10.1007/s11154-022-09765-2

[4] Aitken RJ. Male reproductive ageing: A radical road to ruin. Human Reproduction. 2023;**38**(10):1861-1871. DOI: 10.1093/humrep/dead157

[5] Xia K, Luo P, Yu J, He S, Dong L, Gao F, et al. Single-cell RNA sequencing reveals transcriptomic landscape and potential targets for human testicular ageing. Human Reproduction. 2024;**39**(10):2189-2209. DOI: 10.1093/humrep/deae199

[6] Cappola AR, Auchus RJ, El-Hajj Fuleihan G, Handelsman DJ, Kalyani RR, McClung M, et al. Hormones and aging: An endocrine society scientific statement. The Journal of Clinical Endocrinology & Metabolism. 2023;**108**(8):1835-1874. DOI: 10.1210/clinem/dgad225

[7] Barone B, Napolitano L, Abate M, Cirillo L, Reccia P, Passaro F, et al. The role of testosterone in the elderly: What do we know? International Journal of Molecular Sciences. 2022;**23**(7):3535. DOI: 10.3390/ijms23073535

[8] Ford W, North K, Taylor H, Farrow A, Hull M, Golding J. Increasing paternal age is associated with delayed conception in a large population of fertile couples: Evidence for declining fecundity in older men. Human Reproduction. 2000;**15**(8):1703-1708. DOI: 10.1093/humrep/15.8.1703

[9] Belloc S, Cohen-Bacrie P, Benkhalifa M, Cohen-Bacrie M, De Mouzon J, Hazout A, et al. Effect of maternal and paternal age on pregnancy and miscarriage rates after intrauterine insemination. Reproductive Biomedicine Online. 2008;**17**(3):392-397. DOI: 10.1016/s1472-6483(10)60223-4

[10] Belloc S, Hazout A, Zini A, Merviel P, Cabry R, Chahine H, et al. How to overcome male infertility after 40: Influence of paternal age on fertility. Maturitas. 2014;**78**(1):22-29. DOI: 10.1016/j.maturitas.2014.02.011

[11] Wu Y, Kang X, Zheng H, Liu H, Liu J. Effect of paternal age on reproductive outcomes of in vitro fertilization. PLoS One. 2015;**10**(9):e0135734. DOI: 10.1371/journal.pone.0135734

[12] Setti AS, Braga DPAF, Iaconelli Junior A, Borges Junior E. Increasing paternal age and ejaculatory abstinence length negatively influence the intracytoplasmic sperm injection outcomes from egg-sharing donation cycles. Andrology. 2020;**8**(3):594-601. DOI: 10.1111/andr.12737

[13] Vogiatzi P, Pouliakis A, Sakellariou M, Athanasiou A, Athanasiou A, Colaghis A, et al. Male age and progressive sperm motility are critical factors affecting embryological and clinical outcomes in oocyte donor ICSI cycles. Reproductive

Sciences. 2022;**29**(3):883-895. DOI: 10.1007/s43032-021-00801-1

[14] Begon E, Lefebvre T, Arbo E, Bouée S, Darné B, Jaffré F, et al. Does paternal age affect the live birth rate in donor oocyte cycles? A systematic review and meta-analysis. Journal of Assisted Reproduction and Genetics. 2023;**40**(3):617-626. DOI: 10.1007/s10815-023-02714-1

[15] Begueria R, Garcia D, Obradors A, Poisot F, Vassena R, Vernaeve V. Paternal age and assisted reproductive outcomes in ICSI donor oocytes: Is there an effect of older fathers? Human Reproduction. 2014;**29**(10):2114-2122. DOI: 10.1093/humrep/deu189

[16] Zhu Q-X, Meads C, Lu M-L, Wu J-Q, Zhou W-J, Gao E-S. Turning point of age for semen quality: A population-based study in Chinese men. Fertility and Sterility. 2011;**96**(3):572-576. DOI: 10.1016/j.fertnstert.2011.06.058

[17] Oliveira JBA, Petersen CG, Mauri AL, Vagnini LD, Baruffi RL, Franco JG Jr. The effects of age on sperm quality: An evaluation of 1,500 semen samples. JBRA Assisted Reproduction. 2014;**18**(2):34. DOI: 10.5935/1518-0557.20140002

[18] Johnson SL, Dunleavy J, Gemmell NJ, Nakagawa S. Consistent age-dependent declines in human semen quality: A systematic review and meta-analysis. Ageing Research Reviews. 2015;**19**:22-33. DOI: 0.1016/j.arr.2014.10.007

[19] Lee DM, Nazroo J, O'Connor DB, Blake M, Pendleton N. Sexual health and well-being among older men and women in England: Findings from the English longitudinal study of ageing. Archives of Sexual Behavior. 2016;**45**(1):133-144. DOI: 10.1007/s10508-014-0465-1

[20] Bastos P, Freitas MJ, Gomes A, Vitorino R, Fardilha M. Unravelling the power of omics for the infertile aging male. Current Pharmaceutical Design. 2017;**23**(30):4451-4469. DOI: 10.2174/1381612822666161018155247

[21] Guo Y, Li J, Hao F, Yang Y, Yang H, Chang Q, et al. A new perspective on semen quality of aged male: The characteristics of metabolomics and proteomics. Frontiers in Endocrinology. 2023;**13**:1058250. DOI: 10.3389/fendo.2022.1058250

[22] Jimbo M, Kunisaki J, Ghaed M, Yu V, Flores HA, Hotaling JM. Fertility in the aging male: A systematic review. Fertility and Sterility. 2022;**118**(6):1022-1034. DOI: 10.1016/j.fertnstert.2022.10.035

[23] Kidd SA, Eskenazi B, Wyrobek AJ. Effects of male age on semen quality and fertility: A review of the literature. Fertility and Sterility. 2001;**75**(2):237-248. DOI: 10.1016/S0015-0282(00)01679-4

[24] Kovac JR, Addai J, Smith RP, Coward RM, Lamb DJ, Lipshultz LI. The effects of advanced paternal age on fertility. Asian Journal of Andrology. 2013;**15**(6):723-728. DOI: 10.1038/aja.2013.92

[25] Schmidt L, Sobotka T, Bentzen JG, Nyboe Andersen A, Reproduction E, Society Task F. Demographic and medical consequences of the postponement of parenthood. Human Reproduction Update. 2012;**18**(1):29-43. DOI: 10.1093/humupd/dmr040

[26] Zabak S, Varma A, Bansod S, Pohane MR. Exploring the complex landscape of delayed childbearing: Factors, history, and long-term implications. Cureus. 2023;**15**(9):e46291. DOI: 10.7759/cureus.46291

[27] Janeczko D, Holowczuk M, Orzel A, Klatka B, Semczuk A. Paternal age is affected by genetic abnormalities, perinatal complications and mental health of the offspring. Biomedical Reports. 2020;**12**(3):83-88. DOI: 10.3892/br.2019.1266

[28] Janecka M, Mill J, Basson MA, Goriely A, Spiers H, Reichenberg A, et al. Advanced paternal age effects in neurodevelopmental disorders—Review of potential underlying mechanisms. Translational Psychiatry. 2017;**7**(1):e1019-e1019. DOI: 10.1038/tp.2016.294

[29] Anderson D, Laforge J, Ross MM, Vanlangendonck R, Hasoon J, Viswanath O, et al. Male sexual dysfunction. Health. Psychological Research. 2022;**10**(3):37533. DOI: 10.52965/001c.37533

[30] Bhasin S. Men's health. In: Loscalzo J, Fauci A, Kasper D, Hauser S, Longo D, Jameson JL, editors. Harrison's Principles of Internal Medicine, 21e. New York, NY: McGraw-Hill Education; 2022

[31] Spitzer M, Huang G, Basaria S, Travison TG, Bhasin S. Risks and benefits of testosterone therapy in older men. Nature Reviews Endocrinology. 2013;**9**(7):414-424. DOI: 10.1038/nrendo.2013.73

[32] Rodrigues dos Santos M, Bhasin S. Benefits and risks of testosterone treatment in men with age-related decline in testosterone. Annual Review of Medicine. 2021;**72**(1):75-91. DOI: 10.1146/annurev-med-050219-034711

[33] Tajar A, Forti G, O'Neill TW, Lee DM, Silman AJ, Finn JD, et al. Characteristics of secondary, primary, and compensated hypogonadism in aging men: Evidence from the European male ageing study. The Journal of Clinical Endocrinology & Metabolism. 2010;**95**(4):1810-1818. DOI: 10.1210/jc.2009-1796

[34] Mellstrom D, Johnell O, Ljunggren O, Eriksson AL, Lorentzon M, Mallmin H, et al. Free testosterone is an independent predictor of BMD and prevalent fractures in elderly men: MrOS Sweden. Journal of Bone and Mineral Research. 2006;**21**(4):529-535. DOI: 10.1359/jbmr.060110

[35] Ruth KS, Day FR, Tyrrell J, Thompson DJ, Wood AR, Mahajan A, et al. Using human genetics to understand the disease impacts of testosterone in men and women. Nature Medicine. 2020;**26**(2):252-258. DOI: 10.1038/s41591-020-0751-5

[36] Yeap BB, Marriott RJ, Antonio L, Chan YX, Raj S, Dwivedi G, et al. Serum testosterone is inversely and sex hormone-binding globulin is directly associated with all-cause mortality in men. The Journal of Clinical Endocrinology and Metabolism. 2021;**106**(2):e625-e637. DOI: 10.1210/clinem/dgaa743

[37] Bhasin S. Men's health. In: Harrison's Principles of Internal Medicine. 22nd ed. New York, NY: McGraw Hill; 2026 https://accessmedicine.mhmedical.com/content.aspx?bookid=3541&sectionid=295624829

[38] Matzkin ME, Calandra RS, Rossi SP, Bartke A, Frungieri MB. Hallmarks of testicular aging: The challenge of anti-inflammatory and antioxidant therapies using natural and/or pharmacological compounds to improve the physiopathological status of the aged male gonad. Cells. 2021;**10**(11):3114. DOI: 10.3390/cells10113114

[39] Nguyen Hoai B, Hoang L, Nguyen Cao T, Pham Minh Q,

Jannini EA. Testosterone and aging male, a perspective from a developing country. The. The Aging Male. 2023;**26**(1):2223712. DOI: 0.1080/13685538.2023.2223712

[40] Cai Z, Li H. An updated review: Androgens and cognitive impairment in older men. Frontiers in Endocrinology. 2020;**11**:586909. DOI: 10.3389/fendo.2020.586909

[41] Jørgensen P, Kreiberg M, Jørgensen N, Juul A, Oturai P, Dehlendorff C, et al. Effect of 12-months testosterone replacement therapy on bone mineral density and markers of bone turnover in testicular cancer survivors–results from a randomized double-blind trial. Acta Oncologica. 2023;**62**(7):689-695. DOI: 10.1080/0284186X.2023.2207218

[42] Li J-Y, Li X-Y, Li M, Zhang G-K, Ma F-L, Liu Z-M, et al. Decline of serum levels of free testosterone in aging healthy Chinese men. The Aging Male. 2005;**8**(3-4):203-206. DOI: 10.1080/13685530500356010

[43] Kreiberg M, Jørgensen N, Juul A, Lauritsen J, Oturai P, Helge JW, et al. A randomized double-blind single center study of testosterone replacement therapy or placebo in testicular cancer survivors with mild Leydig cell insufficiency (Einstein-intervention). Clinical Genitourinary Cancer. 2022;**20**(5):404-414. DOI: 10.1016/j.clgc.2022.04.017

[44] White WB, Dobs A, Carson C, DelConte A, Khera M, Miner M, et al. Effects of a novel oral testosterone undecanoate on ambulatory blood pressure in hypogonadal men. Journal of Cardiovascular Pharmacology and Therapeutics. 2021;**26**(6):630-637. DOI: 10.1177/10742484211027394

[45] Barnouin Y, Armamento-Villareal R, Celli A, Jiang B, Paudyal A, Nambi V, et al. Testosterone replacement therapy added to intensive lifestyle intervention in older men with obesity and hypogonadism. The Journal of Clinical Endocrinology & Metabolism. 2021;**106**(3):e1096-e1110. DOI: 10.1210/clinem/dgaa917

[46] Pencina KM, Travison TG, Artz AS, Lincoff AM, Nissen SE, Flevaris P, et al. Efficacy of testosterone replacement therapy in correcting anemia in men with hypogonadism: A randomized clinical trial. JAMA Network Open. 2023;**6**(10):e2340030-e2340030. DOI: 10.1001/jamanetworkopen.2023.40030

[47] Morgentaler A. Testosterone therapy in men with prostate cancer: Scientific and ethical considerations. The Journal of Urology. 2009;**181**(3):972-979. DOI: 10.1016/j.juro.2008.11.031

[48] Wallis CJ, Lo K,Lee Y, Krakowsky Y, Garbens A, Satkunasivam R, et al. Survival and cardiovascular events in men treated with testosterone replacement therapy: An intention-to-treat observational cohort study. The Lancet Diabetes and Endocrinology. 2016;**4**(6):498-506. DOI: 10.1016/S2213-8587(16)00112-1

[49] Siltari A, Murtola TJ, Kausz J, Talala K, Taari K, Tammela TL, et al. Testosterone replacement therapy is not associated with increased prostate cancer incidence, prostate cancer-specific, or cardiovascular disease-specific mortality in Finnish men. Acta Oncologica. 2023;**62**(12):1898-1904. DOI: 10.1080/0284186X.2023.2278189

[50] Khera M. Testosterone Therapy and Prostate Cancer: Risk-Benefit and Individualized Treatment. Cranbury, New Jersey: Urology Times; 2025

[51] Fernandez-Balsells MM, Murad MH, Lane M, Lampropulos JF, Albuquerque F, Mullan RJ, et al. Clinical review 1: Adverse effects of testosterone therapy in adult men: A systematic review and meta-analysis. The Journal of Clinical Endocrinology and Metabolism. 2010;**95**(6):2560-2575. DOI: 10.1210/jc.2009-2575

[52] Wang C, Nieschlag E, Swerdloff R, Behre HM, Hellstrom WJ, Gooren LJ, et al. ISA, ISSAM, EAU, EAA and ASA recommendations: Investigation, treatment and monitoring of late-onset hypogonadism in males. International Journal of Impotence Research. 2009;**21**(1):1-8. DOI: 10.1038/ijir.2008.41

[53] Morgentaler A, Miner MM, Caliber M, Guay AT, Khera M, Traish AM. Testosterone therapy and cardiovascular risk: Advances and controversies. Mayo Clinic Proceedings. 2015;**90**(2):224-251. DOI: 10.1016/j.mayocp.2014.10.011

[54] Vickram A, Dhama K, Chakraborty S, Samad H, Latheef S, Sharun K, et al. Role of antisperm antibodies in infertility, pregnancy, and potential for contraceptive and antifertility vaccine designs: Research Progress and pioneering vision. Vaccines (Basel). 2019;**7**:116. DOI: 10.3390/vaccines7030116

[55] Silva AF, Ramalho-Santos J, Amaral S. The impact of antisperm antibodies on human male reproductive function: An update. Reproduction. 2021;**162**(4):R55-R71. DOI: 10.1530/REP-21-0123

[56] Penzias A, Bendikson K, Butts S, Coutifaris C, Falcone T, Gitlin S, et al. The role of immunotherapy in in vitro fertilization: A guideline. Fertility and Sterility. 2018;**110**(3):387-400. DOI: 10.1016/j.fertnstert.2018.05.009

[57] Ajayi AF, Akhigbe RE. The physiology of male reproduction: Impact of drugs and their abuse on male fertility. Andrologia. 2020;**52**(9):e13672. DOI: 10.1111/and.13672

[58] Haidl G, Haidl F, Allam JP, Schuppe HC. Therapeutic options in male genital tract inflammation. Andrologia. 2019;**51**(3):e13207. DOI: 10.1111/and.13207

[59] Kaltsas A, Dimitriadis F, Zachariou D, Zikopoulos A, Symeonidis EN, Markou E, et al. From diagnosis to treatment: Comprehensive care by reproductive urologists in assisted reproductive technology. Medicina. 2023;**59**(10):1835. DOI: 10.3390/medicina59101835

[60] Wang X, Shen C-L, Dyson MT, Eimerl S, Orly J, Hutson JC, et al. Cyclooxygenase-2 regulation of the age-related decline in testosterone biosynthesis. Endocrinology. 2005;**146**(10):4202-4208. DOI: 10.1210/en.2005-0298

[61] Matzkin ME, Valchi P, Riviere E, Rossi SP, Tavalieri YE, de Toro MM, et al. Aging in the Syrian hamster testis: Inflammatory-oxidative status and the impact of photoperiod. Experimental Gerontology. 2019;**124**:110649. DOI: 10.1016/j.exger.2019.110649

[62] Albert O, Desdoits-Lethimonier C, Lesné L, Legrand A, Guillé F, Bensalah K, et al. Paracetamol, aspirin and indomethacin display endocrine disrupting properties in the adult human testis in vitro. Human Reproduction. 2013;**28**(7):1890-1898. DOI: 10.1093/humrep/det112

[63] Kristensen DM, Mazaud-Guittot S, Gaudriault P, Lesné L, Serrano T, Main KM, et al. Analgesic use—Prevalence, biomonitoring and

endocrine and reproductive effects. Nature Reviews Endocrinology. 2016;**12**(7):381-393. DOI: 110.1038/nrendo.2016.55

[64] Kristensen DM, Desdoits-Lethimonier C, Mackey AL, Dalgaard MD, De Masi F, Munkbøl CH, et al. Ibuprofen alters human testicular physiology to produce a state of compensated hypogonadism. National Academy of Sciences of the United States of America. 2018;**115**(4):E715-E724. DOI: 10.1073/pnas.1715035115

[65] Tvrdá E, Benko F, Slanina T, du Plessis SS. The role of selected natural biomolecules in sperm production and functionality. Molecules. 2021;**26**(17):5196. DOI: 10.3390/molecules26175196

[66] Jeremy M, Gurusubramanian G, Roy VK. Vitamin D3 regulates apoptosis and proliferation in the testis of D-galactose-induced aged rat model. Scientific Reports. 2019;**9**(1):14103. DOI: 10.1038/s41598-019-50679-y

[67] Jeremy M, Gurusubramanian G, Roy VK. Vitamin D3 mediated regulation of steroidogenesis mitigates testicular activity in an aged rat model. The Journal of Steroid Biochemistry and Molecular Biology. 2019;**190**:64-75. DOI: 10.1016/j.jsbmb.2019.03.016

[68] Reiter RJ, Sharma R. Central and peripheral actions of melatonin on reproduction in seasonal and continuous breeding mammals. General and Comparative Endocrinology. 2021;**300**:113620. DOI: 10.1016/j.ygcen.2020.113620

[69] Frungieri MB, Calandra RS, Rossi SP. Local actions of melatonin in somatic cells of the testis. International Journal of Molecular Sciences. 2017;**18**(6):1170. DOI: 10.3390/ijms18061170

[70] Mukherjee A, Haldar C. Melatonin membrane receptor (MT1R) expression and nitro-oxidative stress in testis of golden hamster, Mesocricetus auratus: An age-dependent study. Experimental Gerontology. 2015;**69**:211-220. DOI: 10.1016/j.exger.2015.06.022

[71] Muratoğlu S, Akarca Dizakar OS, Keskin Aktan A, Ömeroğlu S, Akbulut KG. The protective role of melatonin and curcumin in the testis of young and aged rats. Andrologia. 2019;**51**(3):e13203. DOI: 10.1111/and.13203

[72] Akbulut KG, Gonul B, Akbulut H. The role of melatonin on gastric mucosal cell proliferation and telomerase activity in ageing. Journal of Pineal Research. 2009;**47**(4):308-312. DOI: 10.1111/j.1600-079X.2009.00715.x

[73] Wang M, Zhu C-Q, Zeng L, Cheng L, Ma L, Zhang M, et al. Melatonin regulates the cross-talk between autophagy and apoptosis by SIRT3 in testicular Leydig cells. Biochemical and Biophysical Research Communications. 2021;**555**:182-189. DOI: 10.1016/j.bbrc.2021.03.138

[74] O'Brien JH, Lazarou S, Deane L, Jarvi K, Zini A. Erectile dysfunction and andropause symptoms in infertile men. The Journal of Urology. 2005;**174**(5):1932-1934. DOI: 10.1097/01.ju.0000177453.14334.a2

[75] Corvasce A, Albino G, Leonetti T, Buonomo AF, Marucco EC. Once-a-day Tadalafil administration improves the spermogram parameters in fertile patients. Archivio Italiano di Urologia e Andrologia. 2015;**87**(3):210-213. DOI: 10.4081/aiua.2015.3.210

[76] Jarvi K, Dula E, Drehobl M, Pryor J, Shapiro J, Seger M. Daily vardenafil for 6 months has no detrimental effects on

semen characteristics or reproductive hormones in men with normal baseline levels. The Journal of Urology. 2008;**179**(3):1060-1065. DOI: 10.1016/j.juro.2007.10.077

[77] Rago R, Salacone P, Caponecchia L, Marcucci I, Fiori C, Sebastianelli A. Effect of vardenafil on semen parameters in infertile men: A pilot study evaluating short-term treatment. Journal of Endocrinological Investigation. 2012;**35**(10):897-900. DOI: 10.3275/8368

[78] Dimitriadis F, Tsambalas S, Tsounapi P, Kawamura H, Vlachopoulou E, Haliasos N, et al. Effects of phosphodiesterase-5 inhibitors on Leydig cell secretory function in oligoasthenospermic infertile men: A randomized trial. BJU International. 2010;**106**(8):1181-1185. DOI: 10.1111/j.1464-410X.2010.09243.x

[79] Mostafa T. In vitro sildenafil citrate use as a sperm motility stimulant. Fertility and Sterility. 2007;**88**(4):994-996. DOI: 10.1016/j.fertnstert.2006.11.182

[80] Pomara G, Morelli G, Canale D, Turchi P, Caglieresi C, Moschini C, et al. Alterations in sperm motility after acute oral administration of sildenafil or tadalafil in young, infertile men. Fertility and Sterility. 2007;**88**(4):860-865. DOI: 10.1016/j.fertnstert.2006.12.019

[81] Dong L, Zhang X, Yan X, Shen Y, Li Y, Yu X. Effect of phosphodiesterase-5 inhibitors on the treatment of male infertility: A systematic review and meta-analysis. The World Journal of Men's Health. 2021;**39**(4):776. DOI: 10.5534/wjmh.200155

[82] Kaltsas A, Zachariou A, Dimitriadis F, Chrisofos M, Sofikitis N. Empirical treatments for male infertility: A focus on lifestyle modifications and medicines. Diseases. 2024;**12**(9):209. DOI: 10.3390/diseases12090209

[83] Lu Y, Su H, Zhang J, Wang Y, Li H. Treatment of poor sperm quality and erectile dysfunction with oral pentoxifylline: A systematic review. Frontiers in Pharmacology. 2022;**12**:789787. DOI: 10.3389/fphar.2021.789787

[84] González-Corrochano R, La Fuente J, Cuevas P, Fernández A, Chen M, Sáenz, de Tejada I, et al. Ca 2+−activated K+ channel (KCa) stimulation improves relaxant capacity of PDE5 inhibitors in human penile arteries and recovers the reduced efficacy of PDE5 inhibition in diabetic erectile dysfunction. British Journal of Pharmacology. 2013;**169**(2):449-461. DOI: 10.1111/bph.12143

[85] Kun A, Matchkov V, Stankevicius E, Nardi A, Hughes A, Kirkeby HJ, et al. NS11021, a novel opener of large-conductance Ca2+−activated K+ channels, enhances erectile responses in rats. British Journal of Pharmacology. 2009;**158**(6):1465-1476. DOI: 10.1111/j.1476-5381.2009.00404.x

[86] Király I, Pataricza J, Bajory Z, Simonsen U, Varro A, Papp JG, et al. Involvement of large-conductance C a2+-activated K+ channels in both nitric oxide and endothelium-derived hyperpolarization-type relaxation in human penile small arteries. Basic & Clinical Pharmacology & Toxicology. 2013;**113**(1):19-24. DOI: 10.1111/bcpt.12059

[87] Albersen M, Linsen L, Tinel H, Sandner P, Van Renterghem K. Synergistic effects of BAY 60-4552 and vardenafil on relaxation of corps cavernosum tissue of patients with erectile dysfunction and clinical phosphodiesterase type 5 inhibitor

failure. The Journal of Sexual Medicine. 2013;**10**(5):1268-1277. DOI: 10.1111/jsm.12095

[88] Silva FH, Leiria LO, Alexandre EC, Davel APC, Mónica FZ, De Nucci G, et al. Prolonged therapy with the soluble guanylyl cyclase activator BAY 60-2770 restores the erectile function in obese mice. The Journal of Sexual Medicine. 2014;**11**(11):2661-2670. DOI: 10.1111/jsm.12682

[89] Neuzillet Y, Hupertan V, Cour F, Botto H, Lebret T. A randomized, double-blind, crossover, placebo-controlled comparative clinical trial of arginine aspartate plus adenosine monophosphate for the intermittent treatment of male erectile dysfunction. Andrology. 2013;**1**(2):223-228. DOI: 10.1111/j.2047-2927.2012.00046.x

[90] El-Wakeel L, Fouad F, Saleem M, Saber-Khalaf M. Efficacy and tolerability of sildenafil/l-arginine combination relative to sildenafil alone in patients with organic erectile dysfunction. Andrology. 2020;**8**(1):143-147. DOI: 10.1111/andr.12671

[91] Futura Medical. MED2005 Clinical Programme. Guildford: Futura Medical; 2018. Available from: https://futuramedical.com/what-we-do/med2005/med2005-clinical-programme/ [Accessed: 13 September 2019]

[92] Ralph DJ, Eardley I, Taubel J, Terrill P, Holland T. Efficacy and safety of MED2005, a topical glyceryl trinitrate formulation, in the treatment of erectile dysfunction: A randomized crossover study. The Journal of Sexual Medicine. 2018;**15**(2):167-175. DOI: 10.1016/j.jsxm.2017.12.003

[93] Verhelst J, Abs R, Maiter D, Van Den Bruel A, Vandeweghe M, Velkeniers B, et al. Cabergoline in the treatment of hyperprolactinemia: A study in 455 patients. The Journal of Clinical Endocrinology & Metabolism. 1999;**84**(7):2518-2522. DOI: 10.1210/jcem.84.7.5810

[94] AinMelk Y, Belisle S, Kandalaft N, McClure D, Tetreault L, Elhilali M. Bromocriptine therapy in oligozoospermic infertile men. Archives of Andrology. 1982;**8**(2):135-141. DOI: 10.3109/01485018208987030

[95] Schill W-B. Treatment of idiopathic oligozoospermia by kallikrein: Results of a double-blind study. Archives of Andrology. 1979;**2**(2):163-170. DOI: 10.3109/01485017908987308

[96] Sofikitis N, Miyagawa I, Toda T, Harada T, Mio Y, Terakawa N. The effect of kallikrein on human sperm membrane function. The Tohoku Journal of Experimental Medicine. 1991;**164**(1):23-28

[97] Giovenco P, Amodei M, Barbieri C, Fasani R, Carosi M, Dondero F. Effects of kallikrein on the male reproductive system and its use in the treatment of idiopathic oligozoospermia with impaired motility. Andrologia. 1987;**19**(S1):238-241. DOI: 10.1111/j.1439-0272.1987.tb02339.x

[98] Barkay J, Harpaz-Kerpel S, Ben-Ezra S, Gordon S, Zuckerman H. The prostaglandin inhibitor effect of antiinflammatory drugs in the therapy of male infertility. Fertility and Sterility. 1984;**42**(3):406-411

[99] Yamamoto M, Hibi H, Miyake K. Effects of alpha-blocker on daily testicular sperm production and sperm concentration, motility, intraluminal pressure and fluid movement in the rat epididymis. The Tohoku Journal of Experimental Medicine. 1995;**177**(1):25-37

[100] Hibi H, Yamamoto M, Miyake K. Effects of alpha-blocker on sperm concentration, motility, intraluminal pressure and fluid movement in the rat cauda epididymis. The Journal of Urology. 1995;**154**(2):606-610. DOI: 10.1097/00005392-199508000-00079

[101] Gregoriou O, Vitoratos N, Papadias C, Gargaropoulos A, Konidaris S, Giannopoulos V, et al. Treatment of idiopathic oligozoospermia with an alpha-blocker: A placebo-controlled double-blind trial. International Journal of Fertility and Women's Medicine. 1997;**42**(5):301-305

[102] Comhaire F, Garem YE, Mahmoud A, Eertmans F, Schoonjans F. Combined conventional/antioxidant "Astaxanthin" treatment for male infertility: A double blind, randomized trial. Asian Journal of Andrology. 2005;**7**(3):257-262. DOI: 10.1111/j.1745-7262.2005.00047.x

[103] Moradi M, Moradi A, Alemi M, Ahmadnia H, Abdi H, Ahmadi A, et al. Safety and efficacy of clomiphene citrate and L-carnitine in idiopathic male infertility: A comparative study. Urology Journal. 2010;**7**(3):188-193

[104] Ghanem H, Shaeer O, El-Segini A. Combination clomiphene citrate and antioxidant therapy for idiopathic male infertility: A randomized controlled trial. Fertility and Sterility. 2010;**93**(7):2232-2235. DOI: 10.1016/j.fertnstert.2009.01.117

[105] Paradiso Galatioto G, Gravina GL, Angelozzi G, Sacchetti A, Innominato PF, Pace G, et al. May antioxidant therapy improve sperm parameters of men with persistent oligospermia after retrograde embolization for varicocele? World Journal of Urology. 2008;**26**:97-102. DOI: 10.1007/s00345-007-0218-z

[106] Kaltsas A. Oxidative stress and male infertility: The protective role of antioxidants. Medicina. 2023;**59**(10):1769. DOI: 10.3390/medicina59101769

[107] Adamopoulos DA, Pappa A, Billa E, Nicopoulou S, Koukkou E, Michopoulos J. Effectiveness of combined tamoxifen citrate and testosterone undecanoate treatment in men with idiopathic oligozoospermia. Fertility and Sterility. 2003;**80**(4):914-920. DOI: 10.1016/S0015-0282(03)01123-3

[108] Tadros NN, Sabanegh ES. Empiric medical therapy with hormonal agents for idiopathic male infertility. Indian Journal of Urology. 2017;**33**(3):194-198. DOI: 10.4103/iju.IJU_368_16

[109] Crosnoe LE, Grober E, Ohl D, Kim ED. Exogenous testosterone: A preventable cause of male infertility. Translational Andrology and Urology. 2013;**2**(2):106. DOI: 10.3978/j.issn.2223-4683.2013.06.01

[110] Ko EY, Siddiqi K, Brannigan RE, Sabanegh ES Jr. Empirical medical therapy for idiopathic male infertility: A survey of the American urological association. The Journal of Urology. 2012;**187**(3):973-978. DOI: 10.1016/j.juro.2011.10.137

[111] Eleswarapu S, Naelitz B, Jiang T, Muñoz C, Parekh N, Andino J, et al. (181) combination clomiphene citrate and Anastrozole therapy Iimproves semen parameters in a multi-institutional cohort of men with idiopathic infertility. The Journal of Sexual Medicine. 2023;**20**(Supplement_1):qdad060-qdad174. DOI: 10.21037/tau-23-454

[112] Ahmadi-Asrbadr Y, Hemmati-Ghavshough M, Khanzadeh N, Ansari F, Mohammad-Rahimi M. Comparison of the effect of combined therapy of HCG ampule and letrozole tablet with each method separately on the spermogram parameters in the obese men with idiopathic infertility: A clinical trial. American Journal of Clinical and Experimental Urology. 2022;**10**(4):258

[113] Sanchis-Gomar F, Pareja-Galeano H, Mayero S, Perez-Quilis C, Lucia A. New molecular targets and lifestyle interventions to delay aging sarcopenia. Frontiers in Aging Neuroscience. 2014;**6**:156. DOI: 10.3389/fnagi.2014.00156

[114] Hauger RL, Saelzler UG, Pagadala MS, Panizzon MS. The role of testosterone, the androgen receptor, and hypothalamic-pituitary–gonadal axis in depression in ageing men. Reviews in Endocrine and Metabolic Disorders. 2022;**23**(6):1259-1273. DOI: 10.1007/s11154-022-09767-0

[115] Amini S, Jafarirad S, Abiri B, Vitamin D. Testosterone and depression in middle-aged and elderly men: A systematic review. Critical Reviews in Food Science and Nutrition. 2023;**63**(21):5194-5205. DOI: 10.1080/10408398.2021.2015284

[116] Bennett EV, Hurd LC, Pritchard EM, Colton T, Crocker PR. An examination of older men's body image: How men 65 years and older perceive, experience, and cope with their aging bodies. Body Image. 2020;**34**:27-37. DOI: 10.1016/j.bodyim.2020.04.005

[117] Bennett EV, Hurd L, Pritchard E, Colton T, Crocker PR. 'You're part of something bigger': Interpersonal relationships and older Canadian men's body image. Psychology & Health. 2023;**38**(11):1553-1571. DOI: 10.1080/08870446.2022.2030739

[118] Kummer KK, Pope HG, Hudson JI, Kemmler G, Pinggera G-M, Mangweth-Matzek B. Aging male symptomatology and eating behavior. The Aging Male. 2019;**22**(1):55-61. DOI: 10.1080/13685538.2018.1477931

[119] de Souto Barreto P, Ferrandez A-M, Guihard-Costa A-M. Predictors of body satisfaction: Differences between older men and women's perceptions of their body functioning and appearance. Journal of Aging and Health. 2011;**23**(3):505-528. DOI: 10.1177/0898264310386370

[120] Machado AM, Vilaça M, Patrão AL, Pereira MG. Predictors and moderators of quality of life in male users of anti-aging products. PsyCh Journal. 2023;**12**(1):73-83. DOI: 10.1002/pchj.609

[121] Pieczyńska A, Zasadzka E, Trzmiel T, Pawlaczyk M. Physical activity and fitness in white-and blue-collar retired men. American Journal of Men's Health. 2019;**13**(6):1557988319891360. DOI: 10.1177/1557988319891360

[122] Wang B, Li Z, Miao M, Liu X, Wang H, Liang G, et al. The relationship between physical activity and aging symptoms among community-dwelling men aged 40–70 years in Shanghai, China. Journal of Physical Activity and Health. 2015;**12**(1):87-92. DOI: 10.1123/jpah.2012-0439

[123] Seals DR, Nagy EE, Moreau KL. Aerobic exercise training and vascular function with ageing in healthy men and women. The Journal of Physiology. 2019;**597**(19):4901-4914. DOI: 10.1113/JP277764

[124] Hayes LD, Elliott BT. Short-term exercise training inconsistently influences basal testosterone in older men: A systematic review and meta-analysis. Frontiers in Physiology. 2019;**9**:1878. DOI: 10.3389/fphys.2018.01878

[125] Hackney AC. Effects of endurance exercise on the reproductive system of men: The "exercise-hypogonadal male condition". Journal of Endocrinological Investigation. 2008;**31**(10):932-938. DOI: 10.1007/BF03346444

[126] Wehr E, Pilz S, Boehm BO, März W. Association of vitamin D status with serum androgen levels in men. Clinical Endocrinology. 2010;**73**(2):243-248. DOI: 10.1111/j.1365-2265.2009.03777.x

[127] Fallah A, Mohammad-Hasani A, Colagar AH. Zinc is an essential element for male fertility: A review of Zn roles in men's health, germination, sperm quality, and fertilization. Journal of Reproduction and Infertility. 2018;**19**(2):69-81

[128] Rolf C, Cooper TG, Yeung CH, Nieschlag E. Antioxidant treatment of patients with asthenozoospermia or moderate oligoasthenozoospermia with high-dose vitamin C and vitamin E: A randomized, placebo-controlled, double-blind study. Human Reproduction. 1999;**14**(4):1028-1033. DOI: 10.1093/humrep/14.4.1028

[129] Balercia G, Mancini A, Paggi F, et al. Coenzyme Q10 and male infertility: A meta-analysis. Fertility and Sterility. 2009;**91**(6):1937-1946. DOI: 10.1007/BF03346521

[130] Safarinejad MR. Effect of omega-3 polyunsaturated fatty acid supplementation on semen profile and enzymatic antioxidant capacity of seminal plasma in infertile men with idiopathic oligoasthenoteratozoospermia: A randomized double-blind, placebo-controlled study. Journal of Clinical Lipidology. 2011;**5**(6):460-467. DOI: 10.1111/j.1439-0272.2009.01013.x

[131] Young SS, Eskenazi B, Marchetti F, et al. The association of folate, vitamin B12, and homocysteine with semen quality among men attending an infertility clinic. Reproductive Toxicology. 2008;**25**(4):535-543. DOI: 10.1093/humrep/den036

Chapter 5

Understanding Male Sexual Function after TESE or mTESE: A Narrative Review

Athanasios Zachariou, Ioannis Giannakis, Dimitrios Baltogiannis, Aris Kaltsas, Athanasios Zikopoulos, Sofoklis Stavros, Vladimir Kojovic, Agni Pantou, Atsushi Takenaka and Nikolaos Sofikitis

Abstract

Testicular sperm extraction (TESE) and microdissection TESE (mTESE) have revolutionized the treatment of male infertility, particularly in cases of non-obstructive azoospermia (NOA). These surgical techniques facilitate sperm retrieval for use in assisted reproductive procedures (ART) such as intracytoplasmic sperm injection (ICSI). While mTESE improves retrieval rates by targeting active spermatogenic regions, both procedures can disrupt the hypothalamic-pituitary-gonadal (HPG) axis, leading to hormonal fluctuations, including transient or prolonged testosterone (T) deficiency. The resulting hormonal imbalance increases the risk of erectile dysfunction, hypogonadism, and psychological distress, especially in men with preexisting conditions such as Klinefelter syndrome (KS). This chapter explores the physiological and psychological impacts of TESE and mTESE, emphasizing their effects on erectile function, testosterone levels, and mental health. The review highlights alternative strategies, including selective estrogen receptor modulators (SERMs), gonadotropins, aromatase inhibitors, and emerging therapies such as Leydig stem cell transplantation, to preserve spermatogenesis while addressing hormonal deficiencies. This chapter brings together recent research on hormonal recovery treatments and explores the importance of psychological support in managing infertility-related distress. It addresses gaps in the existing literature by offering insights into specific patient populations and incorporating emerging technologies, such as artificial intelligence and biomarkers, into the discussion.

Keywords: TESE, mTESE, sexual dysfunction, testosterone, sexual distress, mental health

1. Introduction

The intricate relationship between advanced fertility procedures and male reproductive health has emerged as a critical area of study within urology and andrology. Among the most transformative techniques in this field, testicular sperm extraction (TESE) and

IntechOpen

microdissection testicular sperm extraction (mTESE) have become indispensable tools for addressing infertility in men with azoospermia [1]. Both TESE and mTESE involve surgical manipulation of testicular tissue to retrieve spermatozoa for use in intracytoplasmic sperm injection (ICSI). While TESE employs random sampling of testicular tissue, mTESE utilizes microsurgical techniques to enhance sperm retrieval rates by targeting areas of active spermatogenesis [2].

Despite their clinical benefits, such invasive techniques can disrupt the hypothalamic–pituitary-gonadal (HPG) axis, leading to hormonal fluctuations with potential consequences for sexual health. Testosterone (T), FSH, and LH—key regulators of spermatogenesis and male sexual function—are particularly vulnerable to disturbances caused by these procedures [3, 4]. Testosterone decline, for example, has been linked to erectile dysfunction and hypogonadism, a condition characterized by insufficient testosterone production with associated symptoms [5]. These effects underscore the need to better understand the interplay between hormonal changes and functional outcomes in men undergoing TESE or mTESE. This understanding is further complicated by findings that unsuccessful sperm retrieval is often associated with greater hormonal and psychological disruptions, including increased prevalence of erectile dysfunction and hypogonadism [6].

Furthermore, there is a relationship between sexual dysfunction and male infertility. Infertile men have a significantly higher prevalence of sexual dysfunction compared to fertile men, particularly in the domains of erectile function, orgasm, and sexual desire. A meta-analysis, which included controlled studies, demonstrated a notable difference in the International Index of Erectile Function (IIEF) scores between infertile and fertile men, highlighting the negative impact of infertility on sexual health [7]. Research underscores the multifaceted burden of infertility, extending beyond reproductive challenges to encompass profound effects on mental health, self-esteem, and marital satisfaction [8, 9].

TESE and mTESE have enabled many men to achieve biological parenthood, but their effects on hormone levels, erectile function, and the risk of hypogonadism remain unclear. This review explores how these procedures influence hormonal balance, particularly their impact on erectile function and the likelihood of developing hypogonadism. Additionally, factors such as baseline infertility status may further contribute to a decline in sexual function after TESE or mTESE. By examining these relationships, this research aims to provide a clearer understanding of the physiological and hormonal effects of these procedures, with a focus on male sexual health. Furthermore, this chapter brings together recent research on hormonal recovery treatments and explores the importance of psychological support in managing infertility-related distress. It addresses gaps in the existing literature by offering insights into specific patient populations and incorporating emerging technologies, such as artificial intelligence and biomarkers, into the discussion.

2. Methods

A thorough literature review was conducted using three major databases: Medline *via* PubMed, Web of Science, and Scopus. The search strategy incorporated specific keywords such as "erectile dysfunction" combined with terms like "post-treatment," "hypogonadism," "azoospermia," "testosterone (T)," "FSH," "LH," "hormones," "TESE," and "mTESE." To broaden the scope of the review, reference lists from relevant studies were carefully analyzed to identify additional pertinent research.

The review focused on studies involving adult males undergoing TESE or mTESE for azoospermia and infertility. Priority was given to research that provided comprehensive details on these two surgical techniques. Eligible study designs included randomized controlled trials (RCTs) and prospective and retrospective studies, with a preference for English-language publications to ensure consistency in data interpretation.

To maintain a clear focus, exclusion criteria were applied. Studies examining sperm retrieval methods other than TESE or mTESE were excluded to keep the review centered on these specific procedures. Research that did not directly address fertility-related complications was also omitted. Additionally, duplicate studies were systematically identified and removed to enhance the accuracy and reliability of the findings.

A narrative review methodology was deliberately selected instead of a systematic review to facilitate a more comprehensive and adaptable synthesis of the literature. This approach allows for a broader exploration of pathophysiological mechanisms, diagnostic strategies, and clinical implications. Unlike systematic reviews, which adhere to rigid inclusion criteria and predefined protocols, a narrative review enables the incorporation of diverse sources, expert perspectives, and emerging concepts that may not yet be extensively examined within a standardized framework.

3. Overview of TESE and mTESE

TESE and mTESE are advanced surgical techniques utilized to retrieve sperm, especially in individuals diagnosed with azoospermia, a condition characterized by the absence of sperm in the ejaculate [10]. Non-obstructive azoospermia (NOA), the main focus of these procedures, poses unique challenges due to its underlying etiology of defective spermatogenesis rather than physical obstructions in the male reproductive tract. NOA, commonly associated with chromosomal abnormalities, hormonal imbalances, or testicular histopathological conditions such as Sertoli cell-only syndrome and maturation arrest, necessitates techniques capable of identifying viable areas of spermatogenesis [11]. TESE, characterized by its random biopsy approach, risks oversampling non-spermatogenic tissue and inadvertently causing greater tissue damage. Conversely, mTESE, guided by a surgical microscope, targets active spermatogenic regions, substantially improving retrieval rates with minimal disruption to testicular architecture [12]. By reducing unnecessary tissue removal, mTESE exemplifies a targeted strategy that benefits individuals with compromised testicular function. This contrast underscores the superiority of mTESE's refined methodology over the more rudimentary TESE approach [11].

The benefits of mTESE are most pronounced in individuals with challenging histopathological conditions, such as Sertoli cell-only syndrome or maturation arrest. For instance, in men with incomplete Sertoli cell-only syndrome, mTESE has demonstrated an 8 out of 11 success rates in sperm retrieval, equivalent to TESE, but with the added advantage of preserving testicular tissue integrity [13]. Similarly, in cases of maturation arrest, where spermatogenic activity is limited, mTESE achieves comparable success rates while reducing potential tissue trauma.

Several factors, including patient-specific characteristics and preoperative hormonal profiles, play a critical role in the success rates of TESE and mTESE. However, success rates remain unpredictable with traditional clinical and hormonal predictors like age, testicular volume, and hormone levels. For example, lower levels of FSH and higher T/LH ratios have been significantly associated with positive sperm retrieval outcomes, emphasizing the prognostic value of hormonal assessments prior to surgery [14, 15]. Larger testicular volumes have also been positively correlated with higher success rates due to increased presence of functional spermatogenic tissue [16]. These findings demonstrate the importance of a thorough preoperative evaluation, including hormonal profiling and genetic screening for conditions such as Klinefelter syndrome (KS), to optimize surgical outcomes [17]. Procedural success is also heavily influenced by technical expertise, further underscoring the necessity of specialized surgical centers for performing these intricate procedures [18]. The interplay between patient characteristics and surgical techniques underscores the multifaceted nature of successful sperm retrieval.

Emerging non-invasive biomarkers such as anti-Müllerian hormone (AMH), TEX101, microRNAs, and proteomics offer promising avenues for predicting sperm retrieval success [19, 20]. Additionally, advanced imaging techniques like high-frequency ultrasound and functional MRI demonstrate potential in assessing testicular structure and function [21]. Recent studies have investigated the role of color-coded duplex ultrasound in predicting sperm retrieval success in men with NOA, though its accuracy remains uncertain. Ohta et al. examined the potential of high-frequency ultrasound to assess seminiferous tubules using detailed B-mode testicular images. Comparing these images with histological samples, they found thar ultrasound offered a stereoscopic perspective due to greater image depth [22]. Certain features, like reduced tubule diameter and visible gaps, appeared to indicate testicular damage and conditions like Sertoli cell-only syndrome.

Studies by Çelik et al. and Karakus et al. demonstrated that in MRI testis evaluation, elevated choline and creatine metabolite signals strongly correlate with successful sperm retrieval [23, 24]. Specifically, choline levels above 1.46 ppm and creatine above 1.43 ppm were associated with high sensitivity and specificity for positive outcomes. Conversely, reduced choline and creatine signals were consistently found in patients with unsuccessful retrieval. MRI, particularly diffusion-weighted imaging and magnetization transfer techniques, has shown potential in evaluating male infertility and forecasting the outcomes of TESE procedures. These advanced imaging methods allow for the analysis of parameters such as the apparent diffusion coefficient and magnetization transfer ratio, which can help identify testicular hypospermatogenesis [25]. Additionally, proton magnetic resonance spectroscopy has been studied as a non-invasive tool for assessing spermatogenesis in NOA patients. Elevated phosphocholine levels were noted in normal testes compared to SCOS cases [1]. Although differences in apparent diffusion coefficient and fractional anisotropy have been observed, no link to sperm retrieval rates (SRR) has been confirmed. Despite these encouraging results, current evidence is limited to small cohorts, and broader validation is needed before routine clinical adoption [1, 3, 4].

Despite advances in surgical sperm retrieval techniques, like TESE and micro-TESE, studies assessing their success often face notable limitations. Many rely on retrospective designs, which can introduce selection bias and limit the ability to establish causality. Sample sizes are frequently small and heterogeneous, making it difficult to generalize findings across broader patient populations [15]. Additionally, there is often a lack of standardized criteria for defining success, with some studies focusing solely on sperm retrieval while others consider downstream fertility outcomes. Hormonal and genetic parameters used as predictors are not always consistent or universally validated [16]. Moreover, patient factors such as age, testicular histology, and prior medical treatments are sometimes underreported or poorly controlled [19].

These gaps hinder the development of accurate predictive models and limit the clinical application of research findings. Future studies could overcome these limitations using prospective designs, larger cohorts, and standardized outcome measures. Addressing these issues through larger, prospective, and standardized studies is essential for improving patient counseling and optimizing outcomes in male infertility treatment.

3.1 Artificial intelligence (AI) in reproductive urology: Predictive models for mTESE and beyond

Artificial intelligence (AI) is becoming an essential tool in predicting outcomes for men undergoing mTESE, especially those with NOA. Recent studies have shown that machine learning models can analyze a combination of patient-specific variables—such as hormone levels, testicular volume, and medical history—to estimate the likelihood of retrieving sperm during mTESE [26]. One study developed a predictive model using an AI platform that required no coding, demonstrating an area under the curve (AUC) of 72.5%, with 85% prediction accuracy in a small validation group [26]. The testosterone-to-estradiol (T/E2) ratio emerged as a significant contributor to prediction, although not statistically conclusive on its own. Another study employed logistic regression models to predict pregnancy outcomes following ICSI with fresh or cryopreserved sperm. The AUCs reached 0.977 and 0.759, respectively. Surprisingly, logistic regression outperformed other machine learning methods, suggesting that simpler models may sometimes be more effective [27]. A third study used a random forest model trained on over 1800 patients to predict sperm retrieval rates (SRR), achieving AUCs of 0.76 (development) and 0.75 (validation). Key variables included etiology, AMH, and testicular volume. The model was linked to clinical pregnancy and live birth rates, providing a basis for personalized decision-making [28]. Another approach integrates AI not only for prediction but also during the surgical process itself, improving real-time identification of sperm in tissue samples through image recognition and reducing human error [29]. Bachelot et al. tested eight machine learning models to predict sperm retrieval outcomes using preoperative clinical data. Among them, the random forest model performed best, achieving an AUC of 0.90 and 100% sensitivity. Inhibin B levels and the presence of varicocele emerged as strong predictive factors [30]. These AI-driven models provide clinicians and patients with better preoperative counseling and could lead to more personalized, evidence-based treatment strategies, improving both decision-making and outcomes in male infertility care [31].

Especially for complex cases, like salvage m-TESE, machine learning techniques have shown great promise in identifying a set of predictors such as associated with successful sperm retrieval, including testicular histology, hormone levels, and intraoperative findings. These predictive models help clinicians estimate the likelihood of success before surgery and personalize treatment plans. Research has also shown that patients with hypospermatogenesis or favorable hormone profiles, particularly lower FSH and higher testosterone levels, are more likely to benefit from salvage m-TESE. Studies using logistic regression and ROC analysis confirm the value of these predictors [32, 33].

The application of advanced computational techniques shows considerable potential in enhancing the ability to predict sperm retrieval success after TESE/mTESE in men diagnosed with NOA. Innovative models utilizing methods such as random forests and support vector machines are increasingly being explored for their capacity to identify relevant biomarkers, support clinical decision-making, and evaluate treatment effectiveness. However, several key challenges remain. These include the need for thorough validation through robust studies, addressing inherent limitations within current modeling frameworks, navigating legal and regulatory complexities in certain regions, and the lack of prospective randomized trials. Furthermore, issues such as small sample sizes and the emergence of novel predictors must be carefully managed. Addressing these gaps presents a significant opportunity to improve diagnostic precision, tailor treatments more effectively, and ultimately enhance patient care in the field of male infertility.

3.2 Ethical and financial considerations about TESE/mTESE

Ethical considerations, cost, and accessibility remain key barriers to the widespread adoption of these innovations [31]. Ethical considerations include informed consent and ensuring patients fully understand the risks, benefits, and potential outcomes. The emotional and psychological impact on individuals and couples must be addressed, especially when outcomes are uncertain. Privacy and confidentiality when handling reproductive material are essential. There are also broader concerns about the use of assisted reproductive technologies, including the welfare of potential offspring. Equity of access to these procedures and respect for diverse cultural or personal values around fertility treatment are important ethical aspects [15].

For men facing NOA, procedures like TESE/mTESE offer a potential pathway to biological fatherhood. mTESE is generally preferred by specialists due to its superior sperm retrieval success, with rates reaching approximately 52%, compared to around 35% for traditional TESE [34]. Despite its clinical advantages, the financial implications are considerable. Data from the United States show that without comprehensive insurance coverage, many patients are left to cover substantial costs out of pocket. mTESE alone can cost between $2500 and $9000, while a single IVF/ICSI cycle may approach $18,000. Adding yearly sperm storage fees, often over $1300, can make this route prohibitively expensive for many couples [35].

Research by Han and colleagues highlighted that among various surgical options, frozen micro-TESE stands out as the most financially favorable. It presents a significantly lower estimated net loss of approximately $9624, representing a substantial improvement compared to the losses associated with traditional fresh TESE approaches. Notably, the study's findings remained consistent across different budget scenarios and IVF-related expenses [35]. On another front, hormone-based medical treatments—especially in men with hypogonadotropic hypogonadism—have shown promise in improving surgical outcomes or even making surgery unnecessary by stimulating natural sperm production. However, for other types of NOA, particularly those with unclear causes or linked to hormonal imbalances, evidence supporting these treatments is inconsistent. Given these challenges, there is an increasing need to improve financial accessibility and develop more personalized treatment strategies that include non-surgical options when appropriate [36].

4. Male erectile function after TESE or mTESE procedures

Despite its advantages, mTESE is not without drawbacks, as postoperative hypogonadism remains a significant concern. A notable example is the development of testosterone deficiency in 13.5% of eugonadal men undergoing mTESE, emphasizing the procedure's potential to induce hormonal deficiencies, even in individuals with initially normal profiles [37]. This risk is particularly pronounced in patients with predisposing factors such as low baseline testicular volume, prior testosterone replacement therapy (TRT), or chromosomal abnormalities [38]. While mTESE minimizes tissue trauma relative to TESE, its capacity to exacerbate hormonal imbalances in vulnerable populations necessitates tailored approaches to both surgical planning and postoperative care.

4.1 Prevalence and causes of sexual dysfunction in infertile men

Sexual dysfunction includes a range of disorders such as erectile dysfunction (ED), premature ejaculation, hypoactive sexual desire disorder, orgasmic dysfunction, and ejaculatory disorders. All males undergoing procedures such as TESE or mTESE usually present major fertility problems. Studies indicate that hypoactive sexual desire and lack of sexual satisfaction are the most common sexual dysfunctions in infertile men, with reported prevalence rates ranging from 8.9 to 68.7% [39]. Erectile dysfunction and premature ejaculation occur in approximately one in six infertile men, while orgasmic dysfunction affects around one in ten [8].

Several psychological and physiological factors contribute to the high prevalence of sexual dysfunction among infertile men. Psychological burdens, such as anxiety, depression, and stress related to fertility concerns, can negatively affect sexual performance [8]. The emotional burden of infertility, including frustration and self-esteem issues, often results in decreased sexual satisfaction. Studies show that infertility-related stress can trigger or worsen ED, premature ejaculation (PE), and hypoactive sexual desire disorder (HSDD) [40]. In some cases, the pressure to conceive during specific time frames (such as ovulation) can further exacerbate sexual difficulties.

Men diagnosed with azoospermia often experience a greater psychological impact, leading to higher rates of sexual dysfunction. The distress of receiving an infertility diagnosis can lead to temporary or prolonged ED, loss of libido, and impaired orgasmic function [41].

Additionally, general health disturbances, including cardiovascular diseases, metabolic disorders, and hormonal imbalances, may contribute to both infertility and sexual dysfunction. Erectile dysfunction in infertile men may also serve as an early marker of poor overall health, highlighting the importance of comprehensive health evaluations in affected individuals [42]. Furthermore, medications used to treat systemic illnesses, including antihypertensives, antidepressants, and chemotherapy drugs, can negatively affect both sperm quality and sexual performance.

4.2 Erectile dysfunction due to post-TESE hormonal alterations

The examination of hormonal changes following TESE and mTESE procedures reveals critical insights into the transient and potentially long-term effects on the HPG axis. A significant decline in T levels has been consistently observed immediately after these surgical interventions, attributed primarily to the disruption of Leydig cell function due to testicular tissue trauma. This decline is typically transient, with recovery generally reported within 12 to 18 months [43, 44]. The immediate postoperative drop in T levels can be substantial; for example, a reduction from 3.81 ng/mL to 3.05 ng/mL within the first postoperative week has been documented [45]. While such changes are often reversible, individuals with preexisting conditions, including chromosomal abnormalities such as Klinefelter syndrome or low baseline T levels, may experience delayed recovery or even permanent hormonal disturbances [46, 47].

These findings highlight the importance of long-term hormonal monitoring to identify and manage any complications, such as hypogonadism, that could adversely impact quality of life [32].

Compensatory elevations in FSH and LH levels are another common postoperative alteration, reflecting the body's feedback response to surgically induced Leydig cell dysfunction and tissue trauma. This rise in gonadotropin levels is a direct consequence of the damaged testicular tissue's compromised ability to produce testosterone, forcing the HPG axis to amplify hormonal signaling in an effort to restore testicular function [17, 32]. The extent of these hormonal changes often varies and is influenced by baseline hormonal levels and testicular histopathology, such as severe conditions like Sertoli-cell-only syndrome [17, 46]. This variability underscores the necessity of individualized preoperative evaluations, with particular attention to FSH and LH levels, as these can serve as predictors of the hormonal response to surgical intervention [48]. Although FSH and LH levels generally stabilize over time as the recovery process progresses, the degree of stabilization can significantly influence long-term outcomes, including sexual health and overall endocrine stability [32]. Compensatory elevations in FSH and LH levels after TESE or mTESE procedures are presented in **Figure 1**.

Patients with lower baseline testosterone levels or genetic conditions like Klinefelter syndrome are particularly susceptible to prolonged hormonal imbalances following TESE and mTESE [47]. Individuals with Klinefelter syndrome, characterized by primary hypogonadism, typically present with elevated FSH and LH levels and diminished T production due to testicular dysfunction [48]. These patients are at heightened risk for developing postoperative hypogonadism, which necessitates proactive management strategies, including preoperative hormonal optimization and genetic screening [49]. While T supplementation has been considered to mitigate the risk of prolonged disturbances, its efficacy in this context remains inconclusive and warrants further investigation.

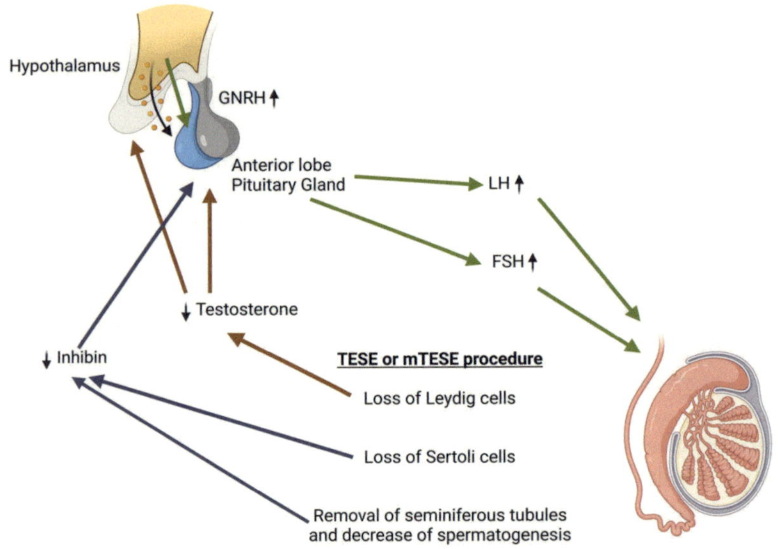

Figure 1.
Compensatory elevations in FSH and LH levels after TESE or mTESE procedures.

Eliveld et al. confirmed that men with Klinefelter syndrome face the highest risk of developing hypogonadism after TESE, with approximately 36% requiring TRT [6]. In contrast, only 3–4% of men with NOA or obstructive azoospermia (OA) develop clinical hypogonadism requiring treatment. The symptoms of hypogonadism observed in men after TESE included reduced energy levels, lower libido, decreased muscle strength, erectile dysfunction, and depressed mood. These symptoms manifest at varying degrees depending on the individual's baseline T levels and their body's ability to compensate post-TESE. In men with Klinefelter syndrome, the drop in T was more pronounced due to their already compromised Leydig cell function [50]. A decline in T levels is directly associated with symptoms of hypogonadism, especially at levels ranging between 8 and 12 nmol/L [51]. On average, TRT was initiated 8 months post-TESE, but cases ranged from 1 to 15 months. Importantly, some men with new-onset low T levels did not exhibit clinical symptoms and, therefore, did not require TRT [6].

Factors contributing to *uncompensated hypogonadism* after surgical sperm retrieval remain unclear. In NOA patients, inconsistent FSH changes may result from scarring, vascular damage, or local germ cell loss. Peritubular scarring may also affect Leydig cell function and germ cell numbers [52]. The differing responses in FSH and LH levels post-micro-TESE suggest that men with typical 46,XY chromosomes may adapt better than those with 47, XXY (Klinefelter syndrome). Research indicates that men with KS may have impaired pituitary responsiveness or a less effective testicular response compared to idiopathic NOA cases [53]. Additionally, extensive tubular hyalinization in Klinefelter syndrome may reduce peritubular scarring, explaining why postoperative FSH and LH levels show minimal variation.

In idiopathic NOA, T levels typically decline postoperatively, reaching the lowest levels around 6 months, with a mean decrease of 78 ng/dL (2.7 nmol/L). Recovery to baseline usually occurs by 18 months, with T returning to ≥93.1% of preoperative levels in most cases, depending on histology (e.g., 93.1% for maturation arrest and 80.6% for Sertoli cell-only syndrome) [54]. In contrast, men with KS experience a more profound and prolonged drop in testosterone. Six months post-mTESE, KS patients may exhibit a mean T decline of 118 ng/dL (4.1 nmol/L), and recovery is delayed, often not reaching baseline until 26 months postoperatively [54]. Notably, only 50% of KS patients demonstrate testosterone recovery at 12 months [54]. In **Figure 2**, there is a graphical comparison of the hormonal recovery timeline in the different patients' groups. In a separate study, 36% of eugonadal NOA patients (TT > 300 ng/dL) developed biochemical hypogonadism (TT ≤ 300 ng/dL) at an average of 26 months post-mTESE. These findings underscore the need for individualized endocrine follow-up, especially for KS patients who have smaller testicular volume and intrinsic Leydig cell dysfunction, placing them at greater risk of permanent hypogonadism [55].

Long-term monitoring of hormonal profiles is essential, particularly for individuals with unsuccessful sperm retrieval or predisposing conditions, to identify and address persistent imbalances and their implications for sexual and overall health. Regular endocrinological assessments enable the early identification of hypogonadism, allowing timely interventions to mitigate potential systemic issues such as osteoporosis or erectile dysfunction [32].

4.3 Psychological reasons for erectile dysfunction after TESE procedure

Research has indicated that postoperative erectile dysfunction (ED) is more prevalent among patients with unsuccessful sperm retrieval following these procedures.

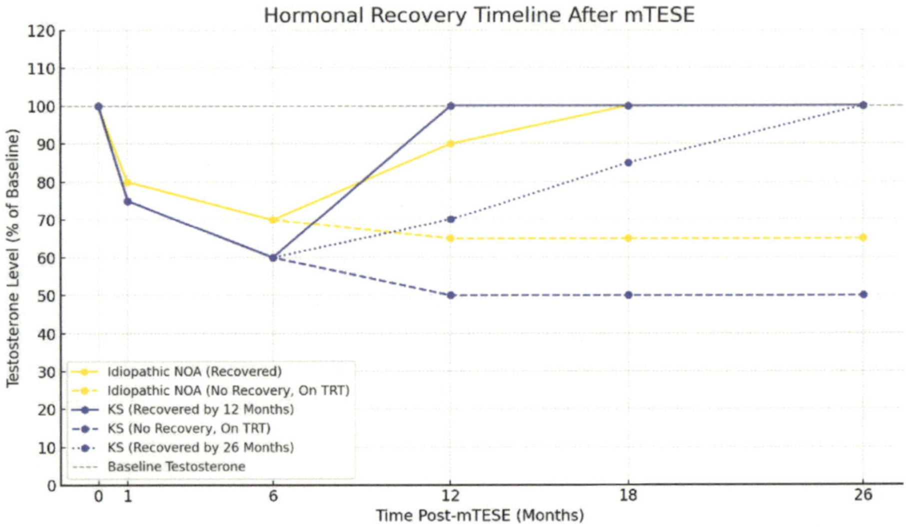

Figure 2.
A graphical comparison of the hormonal recovery timeline in the different patients' groups.

For example, 26% of men in the TESE-negative group reported new-onset ED 6 months after the intervention, compared to only 0.4% in the TESE-positive group [56]. This disparity underscores the significant interplay between TESE outcomes and sexual health. It is evident that the success of sperm retrieval extends beyond fulfilling reproductive goals, influencing overall sexual well-being. Hormonal disruptions and psychological distress following unsuccessful sperm retrieval may exacerbate the risk of ED, suggesting the necessity of optimizing procedural success to safeguard sexual function. Furthermore, the procedural failure likely initiates a cascade of hormonal and psychosocial challenges, necessitating comprehensive pre- and postoperative care aimed at mitigating such risks.

According to Taniguchi et al. sexual activity among patients undergoing TESE remains comparable to that of the general population [57]. The findings demonstrate that factors such as patient age, partner age, testicular volume, and serum testosterone levels do not significantly influence the frequency of sexual intercourse before TESE. The study reports an average sexual frequency of *3.6 ± 2.6 times per month* among patients, indicating that pre-procedural sexual activity does not negatively affect outcomes [57]. Furthermore, *no restrictions or contraindications* were reported regarding pre-TESE sexual activity. The study primarily aimed to assess sexual behavior among patients and identified *marriage duration* as a factor influencing sexual activity frequency rather than any physiological or hormonal limitations. These findings suggest that couples trying to conceive through assisted reproduction techniques can continue engaging in sexual intercourse before undergoing mTESE without concerns of adverse effects.

Unsuccessful TESE and mTESE procedures appear to affect erectile function through interconnected hormonal and psychological mechanisms. Hormonal imbalances, including a marked decline in T levels, stand out as a critical factor. Testosterone serves as a central regulator of erectile function, and its substantial decrease observed in men with new-onset ED highlights its pivotal role. For instance, T levels in patients reporting new-onset ED post-TESE decreased from 7.83 ± 2 to 2.8 ± 2 ng/mL, reflecting the physiological toll of these procedures [56–59]. Beyond hormonal aspects, psychological factors such as anxiety and depression were also consistently identified as contributors to ED, as evidenced by higher Hospital Anxiety and Depression Scale (HADS) scores in men with unsuccessful outcomes [56].

According to Bendayan et al. men who do not have viable sperm retrieved through mTESE often experience *reduced self-esteem, sexual dysfunction, and deterioration in their romantic relationships*. The study found that a negative TESE outcome led to a *significant decline in overall self-esteem*, affecting personal, social, professional, and family-related aspects of identity. This suggests that infertility, when confirmed as irreversible, deeply impacts a man's sense of self-worth. In terms of *sexual health*, men with a negative TESE outcome reported *worsened erectile function, reduced intercourse satisfaction, and diminished orgasmic function* compared to their pre-surgery state. This indicates that the psychological distress of a failed TESE can manifest in physical symptoms, potentially exacerbating *erectile dysfunction and decreased sexual desire* [58].

Additionally, the *quality of the couple's relationship* was significantly affected. Men with unsuccessful TESE outcomes showed *reduced dyadic adjustment, lower consensus, decreased satisfaction, and weakened affection*. This suggests that the emotional strain of a failed procedure can create tension and distance between partners, requiring *strong emotional support and counseling* to navigate [58].

The strong correlation between elevated anxiety scores and ED emphasizes the necessity of integrating psychosocial assessments into the pre- and postoperative care framework [58]. These findings also suggest that the emotional distress following an unsuccessful sperm retrieval outcome is multifaceted, extending beyond sexual health to affect broader aspects of mental well-being. Support systems, including counseling and patient education, could play a vital role in minimizing the psychosocial impact of these procedures. Given these findings, mental health professionals should be actively involved in the care team, emphasizing holistic approaches to patient care that extend beyond physiological parameters.

Several studies have demonstrated the association between successful TESE outcomes and improved sexual health parameters, including erectile function. Men who achieved successful sperm retrieval reported improved IIEF-5 scores postoperatively, which reflect enhanced sexual satisfaction and function [56, 58]. These improvements likely stem from a combination of psychological relief and the maintenance of stable testosterone levels. The psychological benefits of successful outcomes, including increased self-esteem and reduced anxiety, further underscore the importance of achieving procedural success. Furthermore, hormonal stability in men with positive outcomes emphasizes the need for comprehensive preoperative assessments, particularly hormonal profiling, to identify candidates likely to benefit from these procedures [58].

5. The ICSI procedure after TESE

Opting for donor sperm following unsuccessful intracytoplasmic sperm injection (ICSI) can have significant psychological and physiological consequences for men, particularly affecting erectile function. Research by Yin et al. (2024) indicates that men who turn to donor sperm after failed ICSI cycles face increased levels of stress, anxiety, depression, and ED compared to those who persist with ICSI treatments [60, 61].

The psychological impact of using donor sperm often stems from feelings of inadequacy, concerns about losing genetic ties, and societal perceptions, all of which can contribute to psychogenic ED. The study reported that *82.35% of men in the donor*

	Section	Key findings	Supportive evidence	References
1	Male Erectile Function after TESE or mTESE procedures	mTESE can lead to T deficiency even in eugonadal men. High risk in those with low baseline testicular volume or chromosomal anomalies.	Studies show hormonal disturbances post-mTESE, necessitating monitoring	[37, 38]
2	Prevalence and causes of sexual dysfunction in infertile men	Sexual dysfunction prevalence varies from 8.9-68.7%, ED and premature ejaculation occur in one in six infertile men; orgasmic dysfunction in one in ten.	Infertility stress and health conditions impact sexual function	[8, 39–41]
3	Erectile dysfunction due to post-TESE procedure hormonal alterations	TESE and mTESE can cause a significant decline in T, typically recovering in 12-18 months. High risk in Klinefelter syndrome patients.	Long-term monitoring is essential for individuals with preexisting conditions	[6, 43–52]
4	Psychological reasons for ED after TESE procedure	Unsuccessful sperm retrieval increases ED risk. Psychological stress and hormonal changes contribute.	Studies highlight the need for psychological support post-TESE	[56–59]
5	The ICSI procedure after TESE	Using donor sperm after failed ICSI increases stress, anxiety, depression, and ED. Timed intercourse in ART procedures exacerbates performance anxiety.	Research indicates a strong link between ART stress and ED	[60–62]

Table 1.
Key findings about erectile dysfunction after TESE or mTESE procedures.

sperm group experienced ED, a prevalence significantly higher than that observed in both the general population and other infertility-related conditions.

Moreover, the structured timing of intercourse during assisted reproductive technology (ART) procedures intensifies performance anxiety, further impairing erectile function [62]. Timed intercourse was found to elevate the likelihood of sexual dysfunction in both men and women, even after accounting for factors such as age, medical conditions, obesity, smoking, infertility causes, and prior use of assisted reproductive techniques. Men undergoing timed intercourse faced a higher risk of ED, premature ejaculation, and hypoactive sexual desire. Key findings on erectile dysfunction after TESE or mTESE procedures are presented in **Table 1**.

6. The silent aftermath: Long-term hormonal effects following surgery

A decline in T levels after surgery can lead to a range of long-lasting health effects that go well beyond sexual performance. Testosterone is also essential for maintaining emotional balance, cognitive clarity, and physical strength [63]. In men who do not receive adequate hormonal monitoring after surgery, a progressive drop in testosterone is often observed. This hormonal decline may manifest early as reduced libido, fewer spontaneous erections, and, frequently, erectile dysfunction [3, 5].

Over time, insufficient testosterone can contribute to muscle loss, increased fat accumulation, and weakened bones—conditions that heighten the risk of osteoporosis and injury [64]. Mentally, affected individuals often experience chronic fatigue, irritability, low mood, and even depressive symptoms, as well as challenges with memory and focus. These issues may be mistakenly attributed to normal aging or lifestyle factors, delaying proper diagnosis and treatment [65].

There is also a growing recognition of the link between T deficiency and more serious health concerns. Research shows that men with low T levels have a greater likelihood of developing conditions like type 2 diabetes, cardiovascular disease, and metabolic syndrome, highlighting the hormone's broader impact on overall health [66]. Notably, T-related erectile issues can serve as early warnings of underlying heart problems.

From a medical standpoint, assessing T in men with ongoing sexual dysfunction, fatigue, or mood disturbances is critical. When hormone replacement therapy is appropriate and closely supervised, it can help restore sexual drive, energy, and emotional well-being [67]. Still, this kind of treatment is not a one-size-fits-all solution—it requires careful consideration of the individual's health profile. Ultimately, the long-term consequences of testosterone deficiency deserve more attention, as timely diagnosis and personalized care can greatly improve health outcomes and quality of life.

7. Testosterone replacement therapy and alternative approaches to preserve spermatogenesis

Testosterone replacement therapy (TRT) is a widely used treatment for male hypogonadism; however, it significantly impacts spermatogenesis by suppressing the HPG axis. Men who develop hypogonadism following TESE or mTESE procedures often require TRT, but special care must be taken to preserve their fertility. To address these concerns, alternative therapeutic strategies have been explored to boost endogenous T production while maintaining spermatogenesis, particularly in men undergoing TESE or mTESE [68].

7.1 Selective estrogen receptor modulators (SERMs)

Selective estrogen receptor modulators (SERMs) are drugs that act as estrogen antagonists in the hypothalamus and pituitary, increasing the release of gonadotropin-releasing hormone (GnRH) and gonadotropins, thereby stimulating intratesticular testosterone production [69]. Long-term use of clomiphene citrate has been prescribed for men with late-onset hypogonadism as an alternative to TRT.

Clomiphene, commonly used off-label, has shown effectiveness in enhancing FSH, LH, total T, and sperm concentrations. A recent retrospective study confirmed significant hormonal and semen quality improvements in men treated with 50 mg of clomiphene daily, regardless of their baseline testosterone levels. This supports the recommendation to consider SERMs for men with idiopathic infertility and testosterone below 400 ng/dL [70]. However, therapy is not without drawbacks. Up to 17% of men may experience a paradoxical decline in sperm parameters, which may not reverse upon discontinuation [71]. Furthermore, thromboembolic events and potential carcinogenesis remain concerns associated with SERMs, necessitating further research [72].

Additionally, while some studies and meta-analyses report improved pregnancy outcomes with SERM use, others show no significant benefits. These conflicting results could stem from differences in study design, sample size, duration, or patient characteristics such as age and hormonal profiles. Additionally, inconsistencies in how outcomes are measured, including semen analysis and hormone assays, contribute to the variability [73].

7.2 Gonadotropins

Gonadotropin therapy is an effective method for managing hypogonadal men seeking fertility preservation. Human chorionic gonadotropin (hCG) alone or combined with human menopausal gonadotropins (hMGs) or recombinant FSH can restore sperm production. The concomitant use of hCG with TRT helps maintain intratesticular testosterone levels and prevent testicular atrophy [74].

While gonadotropin therapy has shown favorable outcomes in hormone-deficient patients, its effectiveness in normogonadotropic men with idiopathic infertility remains uncertain. A few studies suggest that combining hCG and FSH yields better results than using either alone, especially in severe infertility. However, trials involving normogonadotropic patients have reported mixed findings. For instance, the only placebo-controlled, double-blind study on hCG/hMG in idiopathic oligoasthenoteratospermia did not demonstrate improvements in semen parameters or pregnancy rates [69].

Recent meta-analyses indicate that high doses of FSH may enhance sperm count and motility, though evidence remains inconclusive. Some improvement in sperm retrieval following failed mTESE has been observed after FSH treatment, but findings were not statistically significant [75]. Overall, while gonadotropins show promise in specific subgroups, particularly those with hormonal deficits, their use in idiopathic or normogonadotropic infertility requires further investigation. Cost and lack of consistent outcomes limit their broader application, though combined therapy may hold potential for carefully selected patients [76, 77].

7.3 Aromatase inhibitors

Aromatase inhibitors work by blocking the aromatase enzyme, which converts testosterone into estrogen, thus maintaining a balanced testosterone-to-estrogen ratio. These inhibitors have been effective in hypogonadotropic hypogonadal obese men [78]. While testolactone was previously used for this purpose, it is no longer commercially available.

Both steroidal and non-steroidal aromatase inhibitors, such as testolactone and anastrozole, have been associated with improvements in sperm quality, although their use remains off-label [79]. In a recent retrospective study, men with higher body mass index and diagnosed with hypogonadism or subfertility showed marked improvements in hormone levels and sperm parameters after 5 months of anastrozole therapy, with a 46% clinical pregnancy rate [80]. Despite these encouraging outcomes, the evidence remains limited by small sample sizes and lack of randomized controlled trials. As a result, further research is needed to better define the patient groups who would benefit most and to ensure the safety and long-term effectiveness of aromatase inhibitor therapy [81].

7.4 Selective androgen receptor modulators (SARMs)

Selective androgen receptor modulators (SARMs) are compounds designed to target androgen receptors in a tissue-selective manner, aiming to enhance beneficial androgenic effects while minimizing adverse outcomes. Unlike traditional androgens, SARMs do not convert into estrogen or dihydrotestosterone, reducing risks in tissues such as the prostate [82]. Their selective action stems from the unique way they influence androgen receptor conformation and co-regulator recruitment across different tissues. Several SARMs, including enobosarm and OPK-88004, have undergone clinical trials primarily focused on muscle mass and body composition. These studies have shown increases in lean body mass and reductions in fat mass, with minimal impact on the prostate. However, improvements in physical function have not been consistently observed [82]. While not yet directly approved for male infertility, the anabolic and hormone-modulating properties of SARMs suggest potential future applications, pending further targeted research [83, 84].

7.5 Leydig stem cell transplantation

Leydig stem cells (SLCs) are the progenitors of testosterone-producing Leydig cells and are vital for male reproductive health. Found in the testicular interstitial tissue, SLCs possess the ability to self-renew and differentiate through several stages—progenitor, immature, and ultimately adult Leydig cells (ALCs). These stages are marked by specific morphological changes and the progressive expression of steroidogenic enzymes, with mature ALCs responsible for testosterone synthesis. Therefore, SLC-based therapies have emerged as promising alternatives without TRT limitations [85]. Research has shown that SLCs can be isolated using surface markers like CD90, CD51, or PDGFRA, and they can be directed to differentiate using specific growth factors (e.g., PDGF-BB, LH, and IGF-1) or transcription factors like NR5A1 [86]. Innovations in reprogramming techniques—including CRISPR/Cas9 and chemical induction—have also enabled the generation of Leydig-like cells from fibroblasts or stem cells. Experimental studies have shown that transplanting Leydig stem cells (LSC) into animal models led to restored T production [87]. Research indicates that stimulating aged Leydig cells with translocator protein (TSPO) or transplanting LSCs into the testis can improve testosterone synthesis. While still in the experimental phase, LSC transplantation may offer a long-term solution for men with T deficiency without compromising fertility [88, 89]. Key findings on therapeutic approaches for preserving spermatogenesis are presented in **Table 2**.

7.6 Effectiveness of different therapies

The clinical effectiveness of various therapies for male infertility shows notable contrasts, reflecting the complexity of underlying causes and treatment responses. mTESE, particularly in men with NOA, yields a higher sperm retrieval rate and minimal testicular damage compared to conventional biopsies. Aromatase inhibitors and SERMs show divergent efficacy. Aromatase inhibitors increased T but were ineffective in improving sexual symptoms or semen parameters and even reduced bone mineral density, limiting their clinical utility [90]. Conversely, SERMs modestly improved sperm concentration and morphology, and significantly raised serum gonadotropins and testosterone levels, with a favorable safety profile, suggesting their potential as alternatives to testosterone replacement therapy [91].

According to a meta-analysis of de Silva et al., in five non-randomized studies of interventions SERMS showed an increase in sperm concentration (pooled mean difference 6.64 million/mL; 95% confidence interval 1.54, 11.74, I^2 = 0%), an increase in total motile sperm count (pooled mean difference 10.52; 95% confidence interval 1.46–19.59, I^2 = 0%). In the same meta-analysis, four randomized controlled trials comparing SERMS to placebo showed a heterogeneous effect on sperm concentration. The results were of very low certainty of evidence. Limited pregnancy or live birth data were available. No studies comparing aromatase inhibitors with placebo or testosterone were found [92].

Medical treatment	Mechanism of action	Outcome	Level of evidence	References
Gonadotropins	Replicate LH and FSH function by activating Leydig and Sertoli cells within the testes.	Increase in T, sperm concentration, and progressive motility	High	[69, 74–77]
SERMs	Inhibit estrogen's suppressive effect on the hypothalamus and pituitary, leading to enhanced secretion of gonadotropins (LH and FSH)	Increase in hormone levels, sperm parameters, and pregnancy rates	Off-label use	[69–73]
Aromatase Inhibitors	Block conversion of T to estradiol by inhibiting the enzyme aromatase	Increase in T, sperm parameters, and pregnancy rates	Off-label use	[78–81]
Leydig Stem Cell Transplantation	Regenerative medicine	Enhanced sperm quality and hormone levels, elevated expression of fertility-associated markers, and fertility rate	Off-label use	[85–89]
Selective Androgen Receptor Modulators	SARMs interact with androgen receptors (AR), triggering gene expression and producing selective effects in androgen-sensitive organs.	Increase in T levels	Off-label use	[82–84]

Table 2.
Summary of therapeutic approaches for preserving spermatogenesis.

In a review article, Esteves et al. evaluated hCG combined with aromatase inhibitors, SERMs, or other agents. Of the 16 studies, six concerned case reports or small case series, whereas 10 were cohort studies comparing hormonal therapy (various regimens) versus no treatment in eugonadal or hypergonadotropic infertile men with NOA. Gonadotropin therapy (hCG ± FSH) has yielded improved outcomes in several cohorts [93]. For instance, Shiraishi et al. reported a 21% retrieval rate after hormonal stimulation, compared to 0% in untreated controls [94]. Similarly, Selman et al. found sperm in 22.4% of patients after therapy [95]. Collectively, while all interventions offer benefits, their effectiveness is context-dependent, highlighting the need for personalized treatment strategies based on individual hormonal and fertility profiles.

Leydig stem cell transplantation remains experimental, with no human clinical success rates yet reported, though promising results have been observed in animal models. Overall, hormone-based interventions may significantly improve outcomes in select NOA patients, but further large-scale studies are needed to validate these approaches and integrate them into standard clinical practice.

7.7 Ethical implications of experimental treatments

The integration of experimental therapies like selective androgen receptor modulators (SARMs) and Leydig stem cell (LSC) therapies in treating male infertility raises several ethical concerns, particularly as these interventions move closer to clinical use. SARMs, developed to target androgen receptors with tissue specificity, show promise in avoiding adverse effects on the prostate and cardiovascular system. However, their potential to influence reproductive functions and long-term health outcomes in offspring remains underexplored. This creates a need for caution and comprehensive ethical oversight, especially given the lack of long-term safety data [83].

The most complex ethical considerations arise with the use of LSC-based therapies. Generating Leydig-like cells from stem cells or reprogrammed fibroblasts offers an innovative way to restore testosterone production, but also introduces concerns about genetic manipulation, long-term integration into human tissue, and unintended effects on offspring. Furthermore, ensuring the authenticity and stability of these cells before transplantation is still an ongoing challenge [84].

The integration of artificial intelligence (AI) in male infertility treatment presents a range of ethical implications that must be carefully addressed. One primary concern is the issue of informed consent. Given the complexity of AI systems, patients may struggle to fully understand how decisions regarding embryo or sperm selection are made. This lack of transparency can compromise their autonomy and ability to make well-informed choices. Moreover, the challenge of explainability in AI, particularly in machine learning and deep learning models, makes it difficult even for professionals to interpret the reasoning behind certain algorithmic decisions, potentially weakening trust in clinical outcomes [96].

Another significant issue is the impact on reproductive autonomy. While AI offers enhanced precision and success rates in assisted reproduction, it also risks reinforcing societal pressures on individuals or couples to pursue technological solutions at any cost, potentially leading to over-medicalization. This becomes especially relevant when AI is perceived not just as a tool but as a necessary step toward parenthood [97].

From a research ethics standpoint, most AI applications in reproductive medicine are still in experimental phases, with limited clinical validation. This raises concerns about premature implementation without robust data on safety and efficacy, especially considering the long-term health implications for offspring conceived through AI-supported methods. Additionally, there are concerns about justice and equity in access. Advanced AI systems may be available only in high-resource settings or specialized centers, potentially widening disparities in reproductive care. Ethical frameworks must evolve to ensure these technologies support, rather than undermine, equitable and responsible infertility treatment. Together, these emerging therapies demand careful ethical scrutiny, patient-centered regulation, and transparent clinical practices [98, 99].

8. Postoperative care strategies

Tailored postoperative care strategies, including hormonal and psychological support, are indispensable for mitigating the adverse consequences of hypogonadism in patients with unsuccessful or complicated TESE or mTESE outcomes. Hormonal therapies, such as exogenous TRT, are often required to restore endocrine balance and alleviate symptoms associated with T deficiency [100]. However, the success of these interventions hinges on careful monitoring and individualized dose adjustments to minimize side effects. In addition to hormonal therapies, psychological support mechanisms, such as counseling services, are critical for addressing the significant emotional toll of failed procedures [101]. By integrating these modalities into a cohesive postoperative care framework, healthcare professionals can improve both physical recovery and emotional resilience in affected individuals. Non-invasive monitoring techniques, such as regular blood tests for tracking hormonal fluctuations, further enhance the ability to detect and manage complications promptly [101]. Ultimately, a multidisciplinary approach that encompasses hormonal, psychological, and lifestyle interventions offers the greatest potential for improving quality of life and long-term health outcomes for these patients [100].

Male infertility is a growing concern, with lifestyle factors playing a significant role in sperm health and reproductive potential. Poor dietary habits, obesity, smoking, excessive alcohol consumption, and chronic stress have been linked to reduced sperm count, motility, and morphology [102]. Implementing lifestyle changes can significantly improve male fertility outcomes.

A balanced diet rich in antioxidants, vitamins, and essential minerals—such as zinc, selenium, and folic acid—supports healthy sperm production. Regular exercise helps regulate hormones, reduce oxidative stress, and maintain optimal body weight, as obesity is associated with hormonal imbalances and lower sperm quality. Avoiding smoking and excessive alcohol intake is crucial, as these substances contribute to DNA damage in sperm cells [103–105].

Stress management is also vital, as chronic stress can increase cortisol levels, negatively impacting T production and sperm parameters. Additionally, reducing exposure to environmental toxins, such as pesticides, heavy metals, and endocrine-disrupting chemicals, helps maintain reproductive health [106, 107].

By adopting a healthy lifestyle, men can improve their fertility potential and overall well-being. Early intervention and consistency in making positive lifestyle choices can significantly enhance reproductive health and increase the chances of natural conception.

8.1 The role of counseling or support services

When TESE fails to retrieve viable sperm, the emotional toll on men—particularly those with NOA—can be profound. The realization that biological fatherhood may no longer be an option often comes with a wave of grief, identity loss, and psychological distress. For many, infertility becomes tied to deeply rooted feelings about masculinity and self-worth. This can lead to shame, social withdrawal, and a growing sense of isolation [108]. It is not uncommon for men in this situation to experience depression, anxiety, or a quiet detachment from their partners. The effects of failed sperm retrieval do not stop with the individual; relationships often suffer as well. Communication can break down, emotional closeness may fade, and couples sometimes find themselves drifting apart under the weight of shared disappointment [109].

In this emotionally charged context, the role of counseling becomes especially important. Support from mental health professionals can offer a lifeline—helping men come to terms with the outcome, manage their grief, and reframe their identity in a way that is not solely defined by fertility. Counseling also creates space for honest conversations between partners, encouraging emotional openness that can keep their bond intact [110]. Evidence shows that when psychological support is made readily available, men tend to cope better with the outcome and maintain a more positive outlook on their future. Follow-up sessions, particularly those focused on psychosexual well-being, can be invaluable in addressing issues that may arise in intimacy and self-image [111].

Cultural and regional differences play a significant role in shaping the psychological experience of individuals undergoing infertility treatment. Across the globe, people facing infertility deal with stress, anxiety, and emotional distress, but how they perceive and express these emotions is often influenced by their cultural values, social norms, and community expectations. For example, in more collectivist societies, such as parts of Asia or the Middle East, family expectations and social roles may place heavier pressure on individuals to conceive, especially on women. This added pressure can intensify feelings of shame, failure, or isolation when treatments do not succeed [112]. In contrast, in many Western countries, infertility may be viewed more as a private medical condition, although it still impacts mental health and self-esteem. Studies have shown that individuals from rural regions or with lower educational levels report higher stress related to infertility, possibly due to less access to support systems or healthcare services [113]. In the United States, Black and Latin patients were significantly more likely to feel misunderstood by healthcare providers and to express fears about treatment outcomes, such as side effects or birth defects, compared to White patients [3]. Religious beliefs also contribute to psychological outcomes, as some faiths place great emphasis on natural conception or the sanctity of parenthood, which may heighten internal conflict during assisted reproduction [114].

For clinicians and fertility teams, this means taking a more proactive stance. Emotional care should not be an afterthought. Instead, counseling should be part of routine care, especially in cases where surgical sperm retrieval has failed. Normalizing support, providing clear information about next steps, and validating the patient's emotions and cultural settings are key elements in counseling men and their partners.

9. Future research priorities

Future research in male infertility is moving toward a more personalized and precise medical approach, aiming to tailor treatments based on the biological profile of each patient. One major priority is the use of *in vitro* studies on patient-derived testicular cells to test therapeutic responses before clinical application. This method enables the identification of optimal treatment protocols, minimizing the trial-and-error nature of current therapies and helping avoid ineffective dosing or unnecessary drug exposure. For instance, *in vitro* experiments with gonadotropins like human chorionic gonadotropin (hCG) have shown that Leydig and Sertoli cells respond differently across patients, influenced by age and other factors, suggesting the potential for truly individualized treatments [115].

Additionally, the integration of big data, genomics, and artificial intelligence (AI) is reshaping infertility research. AI-driven analysis of molecular data can uncover hidden causes of infertility and help stratify patients based on genetic, metabolic, and lifestyle factors. This systems medicine approach supports the emergence of P4 medicine—predictive, preventive, personalized, and participatory—ensuring that treatments align with a patient's unique biological makeup and life context. It also promotes early intervention and fertility preservation in at-risk populations [116, 117].

Further studies must focus on the identification and validation of specific biomarkers, the use of biobanks, and the development of decision-support systems powered by machine learning [116]. These technologies offer the potential to drastically improve outcomes by guiding therapy selection and reducing time to conception. Overall, the shift toward personalized medicine marks a critical advancement in understanding and managing male infertility more effectively.

10. Conclusion

TESE and mTESE represent critical advancements in male infertility treatment. However, despite their efficacy in sperm retrieval, these procedures can significantly impact male sexual health by altering the HPG axis, leading to potential hormonal imbalances, including testosterone deficiency and compensatory elevations in FSH and LH.

The transient decline in testosterone observed postoperatively is typically reversible, but certain individuals, particularly those with preexisting conditions such as Klinefelter syndrome, may experience prolonged or even permanent hypogonadism.

The psychological impact of TESE and mTESE extends beyond hormonal fluctuations, significantly influencing mental health, self-esteem, and interpersonal relationships. Men who experience unsuccessful sperm retrieval are particularly vulnerable to heightened anxiety, depression, and diminished sexual satisfaction. These psychological burdens not only affect individual well-being but also place a strain on romantic relationships, often resulting in decreased intimacy and dyadic dissatisfaction.

Given these findings, a multidisciplinary approach is essential for optimizing patient care. Preoperative assessments should incorporate comprehensive hormonal profiling, genetic screening, and psychological evaluations to identify patients at higher risk for postoperative complications. Postoperative management should prioritize long-term hormonal monitoring, lifestyle modifications, and, when necessary, TRT to mitigate the adverse effects of hypogonadism. Additionally, integrating mental health support, including counseling and peer support groups, can help address the emotional distress associated with unsuccessful sperm retrieval and infertility.

Author details

Athanasios Zachariou[1*], Ioannis Giannakis[1], Dimitrios Baltogiannis[1], Aris Kaltsas[2], Athanasios Zikopoulos[3], Sofoklis Stavros[4], Vladimir Kojovic[5], Agni Pantou[1], Atsushi Takenaka[6] and Nikolaos Sofikitis[1]

1 Andrology Unit, Urology Department, Ioannina University Hospital, Ioannina University, Ioannina, Greece

2 Third Department of Urology, Attikon University Hospital, School of Medicine, National and Kapodistrian University of Athens, Athens, Greece

3 Obstetrics and Gynecology, Royal Cornwal Hospital, Treliske, Truro, UK

4 Third Department of Obstetrics and Gynecology, Attikon Hospital, Medical School, National and Kapodistrian University of Athens, Athens, Greece

5 Faculty of Medicine, Institute for Mother and Child Health Care of Serbia "Dr Vukan Cupic", University of Belgrade, Belgrade, Serbia

6 Faculty of Medicine, Division of Urology, Department of Surgery, School of Medicine, Tottori University, Yonago, Japan

*Address all correspondence to: azachariou@uoi.gr

References

[1] Kavoussi PK, Atmoko W, Pinggera GM. Technologies to improve sperm retrieval in men undergoing micro-TESE for NOA. Asian Journal of Andrology. 2024;**10**:4103. DOI: 10.4103/aja202450

[2] Achermann AP, Pereira TA, Esteves SC. Microdissection testicular sperm extraction (micro-TESE) in men with infertility due to nonobstructive azoospermia: Summary of current literature. International Urology and Nephrology. 2021;**53**:2193-2210. DOI: 10.1007/s11255-021-02979-4

[3] Corona G, Maggi M. The role of testosterone in male sexual function. Reviews in Endocrine & Metabolic Disorders. 2022;**23**:1159-1172. DOI: 10.1007/s11154-022-09693-9

[4] Corona G, Torres LO, Maggi M. Testosterone therapy: What we have learned from trials. The Journal of Sexual Medicine. 2020;**17**:447-460. DOI: 10.1016/j.jsxm.2020.01.007

[5] Corona G, Rastrelli G, Vignozzi L, Maggi M. Androgens and male sexual function. Best Practice & Research. Clinical Endocrinology & Metabolism. 2022;**36**:101615. DOI: 10.1016/j.beem.2022.101615

[6] Eliveld J, van der Bles I, van Wely M, Meiβner A, Soufan AT, Heijboer AC, et al. The risk of hypogonadism after TESE in men with various types of azoospermia: A prospective cohort study. Reproductive Biomedicine Online. 2023;**46**:973-983. DOI: 10.1016/j.rbmo.2023.02.003

[7] Liu Y, Wang Y, Pu Z, Wang Y, Zhang Y, Dong C, et al. Sexual dysfunction in infertile men: A systematic review and meta-analysis. Sexual Medicine. 2022;**10**:100528. DOI: 10.1016/j.esxm.2022.100528

[8] Capogrosso P, Jensen CFS, Rastrelli G, Torremade J, Russo GI, Raheem AA, et al. Male sexual dysfunctions in the infertile couple recommendations from the European Society of Sexual Medicine (ESSM). Sexual Medicine. 2021;**9**:100377. DOI: 10.1016/j.esxm.2021.100377

[9] Dong M, Wu S, Zhang X, Zhao N, Tao Y, Tan J. Impact of infertility duration on male sexual function and mental health. Journal of Assisted Reproduction and Genetics. 2022;**39**:1861-1872. DOI: 10.1007/s10815-022-02550-9

[10] Majzoub A, Viana MC, Achermann APP, Ferreira IT, Laursen RJ, Humaidan P, et al. Non-obstructive azoospermia and intracytoplasmic sperm injection: Unveiling the chances of success and possible consequences for offspring. Journal of Clinical Medicine. 2024;**13**:4939. DOI: 10.3390/jcm13164939

[11] Colpi GM, Caroppo E. Performing microdissection testicular sperm extraction: Surgical pearls from a high-volume infertility center. Journal of Clinical Medicine. 2021;**10**:4296. DOI: 10.3390/jcm10194296

[12] Ernandez J, Berk B, Han T, Abou Ghayda R, Kathrins M. Evaluating the quality of reported outcomes for microsurgical TESE in men with non-obstructive azoospermia: A methodological analysis. Andrology. 2021;**9**:1108-1118. DOI: 10.1111/andr.12997

[13] Wang X, Liu X, Qu M, Li H. Sertoli cell-only syndrome: Advances,

challenges, and perspectives in genetics and mechanisms. Cellular and Molecular Life Sciences. 2023;**80**:67. DOI: 10.1007/s00018-023-04798-1

[14] Kim TJ, Koo KC. Testosterone to luteinizing hormone ratio as a potential predictor of sperm retrieval in non-obstructive azoospermia patients. Yonsei Medical Journal. 2023;**64**:433. DOI: 10.3349/ymj.2023.64.7.433

[15] Kaltsas A, Markou E, Zachariou A, Dimitriadis F, Symeonidis EN, Zikopoulos A, et al. Evaluating the predictive value of diagnostic testicular biopsy for sperm retrieval outcomes in men with non-obstructive azoospermia. Journal of Personalized Medicine. 2023;**13**:1362. DOI: 10.3390/jpm13091362

[16] Zhang F, Dai M, Yang X, Cheng Y, Ye L, Huang W, et al. Predictors of successful salvage microdissection testicular sperm extraction (mTESE) after failed initial TESE in patients with non-obstructive azoospermia: A systematic review and meta-analysis. Andrology. 2024;**12**:30-44. DOI: 10.1111/andr.13448

[17] Pozzi E, Corsini C, Belladelli F, Bertini A, Negri F, Raffo M, et al. Role of follicle-stimulating hormone, inhibin B, and anti-Mllerian hormone in predicting sperm retrieval from men with nonobstructive azoospermia undergoing microdissection testicular sperm extraction: A systematic review and meta-analysis. European Urology Open Science. 2024;**65**:3-12. DOI: 10.1016/j.euros.2023.12.001

[18] Greenberg DR, Stanisic AV, Pham MN, Hudnall MT, Ambulkar SS, Brannigan RE, et al. Factors associated with undergoing microdissection testicular sperm extraction among men with non-obstructive azoospermia following evaluation by a reproductive urologist. Translational Andrology and Urology. 2023;**12**:1062. DOI: 10.21037/tau-23-45

[19] Li J, Yang F, Dong L, Chang D, Yu X. Seminal plasma biomarkers for predicting successful sperm retrieval in patients with nonobstructive azoospermia: A narrative review of human studies. Basic and Clinical Andrology. 2023;**33**:9. DOI: 10.1186/s12610-023-00173-5

[20] Kaltsas A, Stavros S, Kratiras Z, Zikopoulos A, Machairiotis N, Potiris A, et al. Predictors of successful testicular sperm extraction: A new era for men with non-obstructive azoospermia. Biomedicine. 2024;**12**:2679. DOI: 10.3390/biomedicines12122679

[21] Lotti F, Studniarek M, Balasa C, Belfield J, De Visschere P, Freeman S, et al. The role of the radiologist in the evaluation of male infertility: Recommendations of the European Society of Urogenital Radiology-Scrotal and Penile Imaging Working Group (ESUR-SPIWG) for scrotal imaging. European Radiology. 2025;**35**(2):752-766. DOI: 10.1007/s00330-024-10964-5

[22] Ohta T, Kojo K, Kurobe M, Numahata D, Tatsuya T, Okada S, et al. Feasibility of high-frequency ultrasound for seminiferous tubule assessment and correlation of B-mode imaging with pathological findings in the testis in azoospermia. Journal of Medical Ultrasonics. 2024;**51**:465-475. DOI: 10.1007/s10396-024-01462-8

[23] Çelik Ö, Hatırnaz Ş, Erşahin A, Başbuğ A, Yıldırım GY, Özener V, et al. Testis spectroscopy may predict sperm retrieval rate in men with non-obstructive azoospermia undergoing micro-TESE: A pilot study. Journal of the Turkish-German Gynecological Association.

2020;**21**(2):70. DOI: 10.4274/jtgga.galenos.2019.2018.0154

[24] Karakus C, Ozyurt R. Correlation between high choline metabolite signal in spectroscopy and sperm retrieval chance at micro-TESE. European Review for Medical and Pharmacological Sciences. 2022;**26**(4):1125-1130. DOI: 10.26355/eurrev_202202_28102

[25] Tsili AC, Sofikitis N, Astrakas L, Goussia A, Kaltsas A, Argyropoulou MI. A magnetic resonance imaging study in etiology of nonobstructive azoospermia. Andrology. 2022;**10**:241-253. DOI: 10.1111/andr.13101

[26] Kobayashi H, Uetani M, Yamabe F, Mitsui Y, Nakajima K, Nagao K. AI model developed using machine learning for predicting sperm retrieval in microTESE for nonobstructive azoospermia patients. Andrologia. 2023;**1**:5693116. DOI: 10.1155/2023/5693116

[27] Jia L, Chen PG, Chen LN, Fang C, Zhang J, Chen PY. Machine learning-based prediction of pregnancy outcomes in couples with non-obstructive azoospermia using micro-TESE for ICSI: A retrospective cohort study. Reproductive and Developmental Medicine. 2024;**8**(1):24-31. DOI: 10.1097/RD9.0000000000000080

[28] Tian R, Zhang J, Xu Y, Liu S, Deng C, Chen H, et al. Predicting microTESE among heterogeneous nonobstructive azoospermic patients: The impact on surgical decision and ICSI. Andrologia. 2023;**1**:4825062. DOI: 10.1155/2023/4825062

[29] Kandil H. Integrating artificial intelligence in surgical sperm retrieval techniques: A narrative review. UroPrecision. 2024;**3**(1):17-26. DOI: 10.1002/uro2.100

[30] Bachelot G, Dhombres F, Sermondade N, Haj Hamid R, Berthaut I, Frydman V, et al. A machine learning approach for the prediction of testicular sperm extraction in nonobstructive azoospermia: Algorithm development and validation study. Journal of Medical Internet Research. 2023;**25**:e44047. DOI: 10.2196/44047

[31] Jamalirad H, Jajroudi M, Khajehpour B, Sadighi Gilani MA, Eslami S, Sabbaghian M, et al. AI predictive models and advancements in microdissection testicular sperm extraction for non-obstructive azoospermia: A systematic scoping review. Human Reproduction Open. 2024;**2024**:hoae070. DOI: 10.1093/hropen/hoae070

[32] Boeri L, Bebi C, Dente D, Greco E, Turetti M, Capece M, et al. Outcomes and predictive factors of successful salvage microdissection testicular sperm extraction (mTESE) after failed classic TESE: Results from a multicenter cross-sectional study. International Journal of Impotence Research. 2022;**34**:795-799. DOI: 10.1038/s41443-021-00487-8

[33] Ghalayini IF, Alazab R, Halalsheh O, Al-Mohtaseb AH, Al-Ghazo MA. Repeated microdissection testicular sperm extraction in patients with non-obstructive azoospermia: Outcome and predictive factors. Arab Journal of Urology. 2022;**20**(3):137-143. DOI: 10.1080/2090598X.2022.2028066

[34] Motawi A, Crafa A, Hamoda T, Shah R, Agarwal A. The andrological landscape in the twenty-first century: Making sense of the advances in male infertility management for the busy clinicians. International Journal of Environmental Research and Public Health. 2024;**21**(9):1222. DOI: 10.3390/ijerph21091222

[35] Han TX, Berk B, Ghayda RA, Ernandez J, Kathrins M. Financial decision analysis based on willingness to pay for surgical sperm retrieval approaches among men with nonobstructive azoospermia in the United States. Andrology. 2024;**12**(2):422-428. DOI: 10.1111/andr.13488

[36] Dasgupta S, Le TS, Rambhatla A, Shah R, Agarwal A. Medical treatment prior to micro-TESE. Asian Journal of Andrology. 2024;**10**:4103. DOI: 10.4103/aja202492

[37] Negri F, Pozzi E, Boeri L, Belladelli F, Corsini C, Cazzaniga W, et al. Short-term hormonal changes following microdissection testicular sperm extraction among men with non-obstructive azoospermia: Findings from a large longitudinal prospective multicentric study. World Journal of Men's Health. 2024;**42**:e17. DOI: 10.5534/wjmh.220198

[38] Fraietta R, Zylberstejn DS, Esteves SC. Hypogonadotropic hypogonadism revisited. Clinics. 2013;**68**:81-88. DOI: 10.6061/clinics/2013(01)oa14

[39] Lotti F, Maggi M. Sexual dysfunction and male infertility. Nature Reviews. Urology. 2018;**15**:287-307. DOI: 10.1038/nrurol.2018.20

[40] Zhao L, Zhou Y, Li L, Wang H, Li R. Sexual dysfunction in infertile men: A systematic review and meta-analysis. Frontiers in Endocrinology. 2022;**13**:938664. DOI: 10.3389/fendo.2022.938664

[41] Leeners B, Tschudin S, Wischmann T, Kalaitzopoulos DR. Sexual dysfunction and disorders as a consequence of infertility: A systematic review and meta-analysis. Human Reproduction Update. 2023;**29**:1-15. DOI: 10.1093/humupd/dmac038

[42] Ventimiglia E, Capogrosso P, Boeri L, Pederzoli F, Chierigo F, Dehò F, et al. Infertility as a proxy of general male health: Results of a cross-sectional survey. Human Reproduction. 2022;**37**:558-566. DOI: 10.1093/humrep/deab277

[43] Althakafi SA, Alkhudair WK, Alrabeeah K, Almannie RM, Alabdulaali I, Alzahrani HM, et al. Serum testosterone levels and other determinants of sperm retrieval in microdissection testicular sperm extraction. Translational Andrology and Urology. 2017;**6**:282-287. DOI: 10.21037/tau.2017.03.57

[44] Boeri L, Capogrosso P, Ortensi I, Miacola C, Cai T, Verze P, et al. Diagnostic and therapeutic workup of male infertility: Results from a Delphi consensus panel. International Journal of Impotence Research. 2023;**35**:1-13. DOI: 10.1038/s41443-022-00576-1

[45] Sertkaya Z, Tokuç E, Özkaya F, Ertaş K, Kutluhan MA, Çulha MG. Acute effect of microdissection testicular sperm extraction on blood total testosterone and luteinising hormone levels. Andrologia. 2020;**52**:e13655. DOI: 10.1111/and.13655

[46] Pozzi E, Boeri L, Capogrosso P, Palmisano F, Preto M, Sibona M, et al. Rates of hypogonadism forms in Klinefelter patients undergoing testicular sperm extraction: A multicenter cross-sectional study. Andrology. 2020;**8**:1705-1711. DOI: 10.1111/andr.12861

[47] Sá R, Ferraz L, Barros A, Sousa M. The Klinefelter syndrome and testicular sperm retrieval outcomes. Genes. 2023;**14**:647. DOI: 10.3390/genes14030647

[48] Zitzmann M, Aksglaede L, Corona G, Isidori AM, Juul A, T'Sjoen G, et al. European academy of andrology guidelines on Klinefelter syndrome. Andrology. 2021;**9**:145-167. DOI: 10.1111/andr.12909

[49] Jayasena CN, Anderson RA, Llahana S, Barth JH, MacKenzie F, Wilkes S, et al. Society for Endocrinology guidelines for testosterone replacement therapy in male hypogonadism. Clinical Endocrinology. 2022;**96**:200-219. DOI: 10.1111/cen.14633

[50] Yamini K, Abdel RA, Homa ST. How successful is surgical sperm retrieval in Klinefelter syndrome? Frontiers in Reproductive Health. 2021;**3**:123456. DOI: 10.3389/frph.2021.123456

[51] Tajar A, Forti G, O'Neill TW, Lee DM, Silman AJ, Finn JD, et al. Characteristics of secondary, primary, and compensated hypogonadism in aging men: Evidence from the European male ageing study. The Journal of Clinical Endocrinology and Metabolism. 2010;**95**:1810-1818. DOI: 10.1210/jc.2009-1796

[52] Zohdy W et al. Changes in testosterone levels following surgical sperm retrieval in men with non-obstructive azoospermia: Systematic review and meta-analysis. World Journal of Men's Health. 2024;**42**:123-134. DOI: 10.5534/wjmh.240129

[53] Billa E, Kanakis GA, Goulis DG. Endocrine follow-up of men with non-obstructive azoospermia following testicular sperm extraction. Journal of Clinical Medicine. 2021;**10**(15):3323. DOI: 10.3390/jcm10153323

[54] Herndon CC, Godart ES, Turek PJ. Testosterone levels among non-obstructive azoospermic patients before and after failed microtese. Fertility and Sterility. 2020;**113**(4):e8. DOI: 10.1016/j.fertnstert.2020.02.024

[55] Ishikawa T, Yamaguchi K, Chiba K, Takenaka A, Fujisawa M. Serum hormones in patients with nonobstructive azoospermia after microdissection testicular sperm extraction. The Journal of Urology. 2009;**182**:1495-1499. DOI: 10.1016/j.juro.2009.06.043

[56] Akbal C, Mangir N, Tavukçu HH, Ozgür O, Simşek F. Effect of testicular sperm extraction outcome on sexual function in patients with male factor infertility. Urology. 2010;**75**:598-602. DOI: 10.1016/j.urology.2009.03.065

[57] Taniguchi H, Matsuda T, Nakaoka Y, Morimoto Y. Sexual activity of patients undergoing testicular sperm extraction. Sexual Medicine. 2020;**8**:30-35. DOI: 10.1016/j.esxm.2019.11.001

[58] Bendayan M, Sais E, Alter L, Fathallah K, Jaoul M, Bosset PO, et al. For patients with non-obstructive azoospermia, the outcome of testicular sperm extraction correlates with self-esteem, sexual health, and the quality of the couple's relationship. Basic and Clinical Andrology. 2022;**32**:3. DOI: 10.1186/s12610-022-00143-0

[59] Herndon CC, Godart ES, Turek PJ. Testosterone levels among non-obstructive azoospermic patients 2 years after failed bilateral microdissection testicular sperm extraction: A nested case-cohort study. Journal of Assisted Reproduction and Genetics. 2022;**39**:1297-1303. DOI: 10.1007/s10815-022-02455-2

[60] Yin Y, Wang K, Xu Y, Huang X, Zheng J, Fan Y, et al. The impact of using donor sperm after ICSI failure in severe oligozoospermia on male mental health and erectile function. Journal of

Multidisciplinary Healthcare. 2024;**17**:21-28. DOI: 10.2147/JMDH.S123456

[61] Wang K, Xu Y, Qin N, Guo Y, Bai J, Li Z. Effect of donor sperm on quality of life in patients with severe oligoasthenosperm after ICSI failure. Journal of Multidisciplinary Healthcare. 2025;**18**:123-132. DOI: 10.2147/JMDH.S234567

[62] Dasgupta S, Frodsham LC, Yap TL, Patra P, Chanda A. The negative impact of timed intercourse in infertile couples: A prospective cohort study. Journal of Clinical Urology. 2024;**17**:607-615. DOI: 10.1177/20514158211012345

[63] Theodorakis N, Feretzakis G, Vamvakou G, Verykios VS, Polymeris A, Nikolaou M. Testosterone therapy for functional hypogonadism in middle-aged and elderly males: Current evidence and future perspectives. Hormones. 2024;**1**:17. DOI: 10.1007/s42000-024-00587-2

[64] Oduwegwu E, Kalhan A. Male hypogonadism and osteoporosis: A systematic review. Journal of Endocrinology and Metabolism Research. 2022;**3**(1):1-40. DOI: 10.26502/fjemr.2644-2791.0075

[65] Indirli R, Lanzi V, Arosio M, Mantovani G, Ferrante E. The association of hypogonadism with depression and its treatments. Frontiers in Endocrinology. 2023;**14**:1198437. DOI: 10.3389/fendo.2023.1198437

[66] Oguz A, Sahin M, Ulgen C, Uyan M, Gul K. Overt hypogonadism is a cardiovascular risk factor in type 2 diabetic males: An observational study. Andrologia. 2022;**54**(1):e14271. DOI: 10.1111/and.14271

[67] Wang C, Swerdloff RS. Testosterone replacement therapy in hypogonadal men. Endocrinology and Metabolism Clinics. 2022;**51**(1):77-98. DOI: 10.1016/j.ecl.2021.11.005

[68] Majzoub A, Sabanegh E Jr. Testosterone replacement in the infertile man. Translational Andrology and Urology. 2016;**5**:859-865. DOI: 10.21037/tau.2016.08.12

[69] Kaltsas A, Zachariou A, Dimitriadis F, Chrisofos M, Sofikitis N. Empirical treatments for male infertility: A focus on lifestyle modifications and medicines. Diseases. 2024;**12**:209. DOI: 10.3390/diseases12090209

[70] Delu A, Kiltz RJ, Kuznetsov VA, Trussell JC. Clomiphene citrate improved testosterone and sperm concentration in hypogonadal males. Systems Biology in Reproductive Medicine. 2020;**66**:364-369

[71] Gundewar T, Kuchakulla M, Ramasamy R. A paradoxical decline in semen parameters in men treated with clomiphene citrate: A systematic review. Andrologia. 2021;**53**:e13848

[72] Alkandari MH, Zini A. Medical management of non-obstructive azoospermia: A systematic review. Arab Journal of Urology. 2021;**19**:215-220. DOI: 10.1080/2090598X.2021.1924046

[73] Abdulkareem AO, Tiwari P, Lone ZR, Iqbal H, Gupta S, Jha RK, et al. Ormeloxifene, a selective estrogen receptor modulator, protects against pulmonary hypertension. European Journal of Pharmacology. 2023;**943**:175558. DOI: 10.1016/j.ejphar.2023.175558

[74] Cirigliano L, Falcone M, Gül M, Preto M, Ceruti C, Plamadeala N, et al. Onco-TESE (testicular sperm extraction): Insights from a tertiary center and comprehensive literature analysis. Medicina (Kaunas, Lithuania).

2023;**59**:1226. DOI: 10.3390/medicina59071226

[75] Cannarella R, La Vignera S, Condorelli RA, Mongioi LM, Calogero AE. FSH dosage effect on conventional sperm parameters: A meta-analysis of randomized controlled studies. Asian Journal of Andrology. 2020;**22**:309-316. DOI: 10.4103/aja.aja_42_19

[76] Verdi A, Nasr-Esfahani MH, Forouzanfar M, Tavalaee M. The effect of recombinant human follicle-stimulating hormone on sperm quality, chromatin status and clinical outcomes of infertile oligozoospermic men candidate for intracytoplasmic sperm injection: A randomized clinical trial. International Journal of Fertility and Sterility. 2021;**15**:1-7. DOI: 10.22074/ijfs.2021.135135

[77] Boeri L, Capogrosso P, Salonia A. Gonadotropin treatment for the male hypogonadotropic hypogonadism. Current Pharmaceutical Design. 2021;**27**:2775-2783. DOI: 10.2174/1381612826666200523175806

[78] Sayyad NB, Sabale PM, Umare MD, Bajaj KK. Aromatase inhibitors: Development and current perspectives. Indian Journal of Pharmaceutical Education And Research. 2022;**56**:311-320. DOI: 10.5530/ijper.56.2.51

[79] Del Giudice F, Busetto GM, De Berardinis E, Sperduti I, Ferro M, Maggi M, et al. A systematic review and meta-analysis of clinical trials implementing aromatase inhibitors to treat male infertility. Asian Journal of Andrology. 2020;**22**:360-367. DOI: 10.4103/aja.aja_73_19

[80] Shah T, Nyirenda T, Shin D. Efficacy of anastrozole in the treatment of hypogonadal, subfertile men with body mass index ≥25 kg/m^2. Translational Andrology and Urology. 2021;**10**:1222-1228. DOI: 10.21037/tau-20-919

[81] Yang C, Li P, Li Z. Clinical application of aromatase inhibitors to treat male infertility. Human Reproduction Update. 2022;**28**:30-50. DOI: 10.1093/humupd/dmab036

[82] Neil D, Clark RV, Magee M, et al. GSK2881078, a SARM, produces dose dependent increases in lean mass in healthy older men and women. The Journal of Clinical Endocrinology and Metabolism. 2018;**103**(9):3215-3224. DOI: 10.1210/jc.2017-02644

[83] Kang J, Chen R, Tharakan T, Minhas S. Novel androgen therapies including selective androgen receptor modulators. Best Practice & Research. Clinical Endocrinology & Metabolism. 2022;**36**:101686. DOI: 10.1016/j.beem.2022.101686

[84] Sigalos JT, Walker DT, Lipshultz LI. Selective androgen receptor modulators in the treatment of hypogonadism and men's health. In: Lipshultz LI, Pastuszak AW, Girardi N, Khera M, editors. Men's Reproductive and Sexual Health throughout the Lifespan: An Integrated Approach to Fertility, Sexual Function, and Vitality. New York: Springer; 2023. p. 264

[85] Liu ZJ, Liu YH, Huang SY, Zang ZJ. Insights into the regulation on proliferation and differentiation of stem Leydig cells. Stem Cell Reviews and Reports. 2021;**17**(5):1521-1533. DOI: 10.1007/s12015-021-10133-x

[86] Li ZH, Lu JD, Li SJ, Chen HL, Su ZJ. Generation of Leydig-like cells: Approaches, characterization, and challenges. Asian Journal of Andrology. 2022;**24**(4):335-344. DOI: 10.4103/aja202323

[87] Modanlou M, Mahdipour M, Mobarak H. Effectiveness of stem cell therapy for male infertility restoration: A systematic review. Journal of Investigative Medicine. 2025;**73**:229-252. DOI: 10.1177/10815589241305317

[88] Li L, Papadopoulos V. Advances in stem cell research for the treatment of primary hypogonadism. Nature Reviews. Urology. 2021;**18**:487-507. DOI: 10.1038/s41585-021-00468-0

[89] Sagaradze G, Monakova A, Basalova N, Popov V, Balabanyan V, Efimenko A. Regenerative medicine for male infertility: A focus on stem cell niche injury models. Biomedical Journal. 2022;**45**:607-614. DOI: 10.1016/j.bj.2022.01.002

[90] Awouters M, Vanderschueren D, Antonio L. Aromatase inhibitors and selective estrogen receptor modulators: Unconventional therapies for functional hypogonadism? Andrology. 2020;**8**(6):1590-1597. DOI: 10.1111/andr.12725

[91] Cannarella R, Condorelli RA, Mongioì LM, Barbagallo F, Calogero AE, La Vignera S. Effects of the selective estrogen receptor modulators for the treatment of male infertility: A systematic review and meta-analysis. Expert Opinion on Pharmacotherapy. 2019;**20**(12):1517-1525. DOI: 10.1080/14656566.2019.1615057

[92] de Silva NL, Dissanayake H, Suarez C, Wickramarachchi RE, Ramasamy R, Dhillo WS, et al. Effect of oestrogen modulation on semen parameters in men with secondary hypogonadism: Systematic review and meta analysis. Andrology. 2024;**12**(2):259-276. DOI: 10.1111/andr.13480

[93] Esteves SC, Viana MC, Achermann AP, Santi D. Human chorionic gonadotropin based clinical treatments for infertile men with nonobstructive azoospermia. Andrology. 2025. DOI: 10.1111/andr.70003

[94] Shiraishi K, Ishikawa T, Watanabe N, Iwamoto T, Matsuyama H. Salvage hormonal therapy after failed microdissection testicular sperm extraction: A multiinstitutional prospective study. International Journal of Urology. 2016;**23**(6):496-500. DOI: 10.1111/iju.13076

[95] Selman H, De Santo M, Sterzik K, Cipollone G, Aragona C, El-Danasouri I. Rescue of spermatogenesis arrest in azoospermic men after long-term gonadotropin treatment. Fertility and Sterility. 2006;**86**(2):466-468. DOI: 10.1016/j.fertnstert.2005.12.055

[96] Tamir S. Artificial intelligence in human reproduction: Charting the ethical debate over AI in IVF. AI and Ethics. 2023;**3**(3):947-961. DOI: 10.1007/s43681-022-00216-x

[97] Rolfes V, Bittner U, Gerhards H, Krüssel J-S, Fehm T, Ranisch R, et al. Artificial intelligence in reproductive medicinean ethical perspective. Geburtshilfe und Frauenheilkunde. 2023;**83**(01):106-115. DOI: 10.1055/a-1866-2792

[98] Medenica S, Zivanovic D, Batkoska L, Marinelli S, Basile G, Perino A, et al. The future is coming: Artificial intelligence in the treatment of infertility could improve assisted reproduction outcomes the value of regulatory frameworks. Diagnostics. 2022;**12**(12):2979. DOI: 10.3390/diagnostics12122979

[99] Mills C, Johnston M, Koplin J. Artificial intelligence for embryo selection: Ethical, social and regulatory issues. Human Reproduction.

2023;**38**:dead093-266. DOI: 10.1093/humrep/dead093.266

[100] Binsaleh S, Alhajeri D, Madbouly K. Microdissection testicular sperm extraction in men with nonobstructive azoospermia. Urology Annals. 2017;**9**:136-140. DOI: 10.4103/UA.UA_127_16

[101] Taniguchi H, Shimada S, Kinoshita H. Testosterone therapy for late-onset hypogonadism improves erectile function. Urologia Internationalis. 2022;**106**:539-552. DOI: 10.1159/000521586

[102] Bold J, Swinburne D. Pre-conceptual guidelines for men: A review of male infertility experience, including nutrition and lifestyle factors. Dietetics. 2022;**1**:164-181. DOI: 10.3390/dietetics1030014

[103] Okonofua FE, Ntoimo LFC, Omonkhua A, Ayodeji O, Olafusi C, Unuabonah E, et al. Causes and risk factors for male infertility: A scoping review of published studies. International Journal of General Medicine. 2022;**15**:5985-5997. DOI: 10.2147/IJGM.S378932

[104] Rotimi DE, Singh SK. Implications of lifestyle factors on male reproductive health. JBRA Assisted Reproduction. 2024;**28**:320. DOI: 5935/1518-0557.20220095

[105] Osadchuk LV, Osadchuk AV. Individual lifestyle and male fertility. Human Physiology. 2023;**49**:196-207. DOI: 10.1134/S036211972302012X

[106] Emokpae MA, Brown SI. Effects of lifestyle factors on fertility: Practical recommendations for modification. Reproduction and Fertility. 2021;**2**:R13-R26. DOI: 10.1530/RAF-20-0017

[107] Eisenberg ML, Esteves SC, Lamb DJ, Hotaling JM, Giwercman A, Hwang K, et al. Male infertility. Nature Reviews. Disease Primers. 2023;**9**:49. DOI: 10.1038/s41572-023-00434-9

[108] Wu W, La J, Schubach KM, Lantsberg D, Katz DJ. Psychological, social, and sexual challenges affecting men receiving male infertility treatment: A systematic review and implications for clinical care. Asian Journal of Andrology. 2023;**25**(4):448-453. DOI: 10.4103/aja2022.83

[109] Sharma A, Shrivastava D, Sharma A IV. Psychological problems related to infertility. Cureus. 2022;**14**(10):e30705. DOI: 10.7759/cureus.30705

[110] Iordachescu DA, Gica C, Vladislav EO, Panaitescu AM, Peltecu G, Furtuna ME, et al. Emotional disorders, marital adaptation and the moderating role of social support for couples under treatment for infertility. Ginekologia Polska. 2021;**92**(2):98-104. DOI: 10.5603/GP.a2020.0171

[111] Hamzehgardeshi Z, Khalilian A, Peyvandi S, Elyasi F, Kalantari F, Gelehkolaee KS. Complex factors related to marital and sexual satisfaction among couples undergoing infertility treatment: A cross-sectional study. Heliyon. 2023;**9**(4). DOI: 10.1016/j.heliyon.2023.e14768

[112] Braverman AM, Davoudian T, Levin IK, Bocage A, Wodoslawsky S. Depression, anxiety, quality of life, and infertility: A global lens on the last decade of research. Fertility and Sterility. 2024;**121**(3):379-383. DOI: 10.1016/j.fertnstert.2023.12.006

[113] Galic I, Swanson A, Warren C, Negris O, Bozen A, Brown D, et al. Infertility in the Midwest: Perceptions and attitudes of current treatment.

American Journal of Obstetrics and Gynecology. 2021;**225**(1):61e1-61e7. DOI: 10.1016/j.ajog.2021.02.011

[114] Lei A, You H, Luo B, Ren J. The associations between infertility-related stress, family adaptability and family cohesion in infertile couples. Scientific Reports. 2021;**11**(1):24220. DOI: 10.1038/s41598-021-03719-7

[115] Zampieri N, Camoglio FS, Dando I. A new frontier in therapy personalisation based on *in vitro* studies to preserve fertility potential of men. Andrologia. 2022;**54**(1):e14244. DOI: 10.1111/and.14244

[116] de Santiago I, Polanski L. Data-driven medicine in the diagnosis and treatment of infertility. Journal of Clinical Medicine. 2022;**11**(21):6426. DOI: 10.3390/jcm11216426

[117] Podgrajsek R, Hodzic A, Stimpfel M, Kunej T, Peterlin B. Insight into the complexity of male infertility: A multi-omics review. Systems Biology in Reproductive Medicine. 2024;**70**(1):73-90. DOI: 10.1080/19396368.2023.2253890